Anyone Can Intubate

2nd Edition

Christine E. Whitten, MD

Assistant Chief of Anesthesia
Kaiser Permanente Hospital, San Diego, California

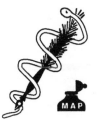

Medical Arts Publications
A Division of K-W Publications
San Diego, California

Ordering Information

Additional copies of this book may be purchased at your local bookstore specializing in professional or medical books or directly from the publisher at the address below. Remit $16.95, paperback; $22.95 hardcover, plus $2.00 for postage and handling. California residents add 7% sales tax.

For information concerning bulk purchases or course adoptions write or call:

Medical Arts Publications
11532 Alkaid Drive
San Diego, California 92126 - 1370
619-566-6489 (8 a.m. - 5 p.m., Pacific Coast Time

Design by Michael D. Kelly, K-W Publishing Services
11532 Alkaid Dr., San Diego, CA 92126

Library of Congress Catalog Card Number: 88-83002

Softcover: ISBN 0-929894-03-0
Hardcover: ISBN 0-929894-04-9

Printing History: 1st Edition published Jan. 1989, 2d ed. Jan. 1990.

Printed in the United States of America
10 9 8 7 6 5 4 3 2 1

Attention Educators

The following instructional aids complement *Anyone Can Intubate* and are available from the publisher.

Teacher's Guide — Chapter by chapter teaching suggestions and 4 multiple-choice k-style tests, **free** to adopting institutions.

Transparencies — A set of more than 65 illustrated transparencies based on the book's *illustrations*. $94.95 per set, with a 10% discount to institutions that adopt the book ($84.45). The transparencies are available by themselves. Write for a free sample.

Slides, color — write for details.

Video — write for details.

CEU credit — Available through Kaiser Permanente, Nursing Education Office. You do not have to be a resident of California to receive this credit. Write or call **619-528-6133** for details.

What readers and reviewers are saying about *Anyone Can Intubate (1st Ed.):*

"... this is a superb handbook for those needing to acquire the skills of tracheal intubation and I shall certainly include it in our basic instruction system for medical undergraduates . . . The literary style is chatty and engaging while retaining the authority of an experienced professional . . . Dr. Whitten takes us through well illustrated airway anatomy, equipment, techniques and complications. She includes a sensible discussion on general airway management and basic ventilation, leading eventually to the handling of the crisis situation by needle crico-thyrotomy. The sections on common errors and difficult intubations are most valuable for the trainee. The line drawings are well placed within the text and are a prime asset of the book."

T. Hilary Howells
British Journal of Anaesthesia

"... and as a {pediatric} MD in private practice who does mainly office medical work this was a needed book for me. . . . I love the author's non-incriminatory approach to those handling emergencies. She knows some of us are apprehensive."

Walter C. Wrobel, MD
Arlington Heights, IL

— over —

Contents

Acknowledgements

No book is ever written alone. I wish to express my deep appreciation for all the help and constructive criticism. I especially wish to thank Doctors Clyde Jones, Anne Wong, James Crawford, Susan Dickerson, and Michael Dickerson for their technical reviews and support. Special thanks to my husband Michael D. Kelly whose inspiration and expert knowledge in editing, design, and computers made this book possible.

To Our Readers

Just as this edition required the help of interested professionals, so too will future editions of this and other Medical Arts Press titles. We invite our readers to read the special note "To Our Readers" on page x of this book.

To my parents
Ward and Bettye Whitten
— for all the years of
encouragement and belief.

To Our Readers

Medical Arts Press is interested in your comments and suggestions. We want to improve this book in any way possible in future printings and welcome your feedback. Have you tips or techniques you'd like to tell us about? If we include them in future editions we'll recognize your contribution.

Please direct your correspondence to:

Dr. Christine E. Whitten
Medical Arts Press
11532 Alkaid Dr.
San Diego, CA 92126

In addition, if there are topics you would like to see treated in future Medical Arts Press books let us know your suggestions.

We will also accept manuscripts for review for subjects in the medical field. Please write to the publisher at the above address.

If you would like to be notified of future editions of this or other Medical Arts Publication titles or teachers training aids please fill out and send in the coupon below to:

Medical Arts Publications, 11532 Alkaid Dr., San Diego, Ca. 92126

- -

Name _____

Address _____

City_____ State_____ Zip_____

Phone (   ) _____

❏ Please notify me of new editions and titles.

❏ Attached you'll find my comments and suggestions.

Introduction

To intubate means to place an endotracheal tube into the trachea. It's a lifesaving skill. Hospitals today expect most doctors, nurses, medical students, nursing students, paramedics, and respiratory technicians to be able to ventilate and intubate any patient.

I've trained many people to intubate in my career as an anesthesiologist. The literature available to learn the basic technique of intubation is very limited. Most texts discuss intubation with the expert in mind. They give a short description of technique accompanied by one or two pictures of the head in cross-section. They lack detailed instruction because intubation has been a skill passed from mentor to student by long apprenticeship. Today's increasing emphasis on teaching large numbers of students the technique during short training sessions requires a different type of textbook. My book is designed to fill that need.

Anyone Can Intubate starts with the essential airway anatomy. With words and pictures you learn how to manipulate airway anatomy

1

in order to intubate. You'll find step-by-step instruction on how to place your hands, move the head, and handle the instruments in a safe and effective manner. You'll learn why each move is important and what it accomplishes. This makes the technique easier to master and it puts you in control. Heavy reliance on illustrations makes visualizing the steps of intubation easier.

Anyone Can Intubate won't replace hands-on experience and practice with a mannequin. However, it *will* tell you how intubating the mannequin differs from the real patient, something often skipped in the short courses. This difference often startles and hinders the beginning intubator the first time he or she makes the transition to a patient..

In addition to routine adult intubation we'll also look at pediatric intubation. Since children's anatomy is different, intubating pediatric patients is different. You'll also learn:

- how to alter your technique when faced with a challenging or difficult intubation,

- steps to take if you cannot intubate the patient,

- strategies for managing the airway during cardiac arrests and other emergencies.

The ability to ventilate the patient is equally important, if not more important, to understand. In chapter 10 we'll discuss how to effectively use a bag and mask apparatus and offer tips for treating airway obstruction.

Anyone Can Intubate gives you a visual picture of intubation. As you proceed through the book, picture yourself performing the steps. Understand why moving the patient's head in a certain way, or changing the angle of your laryngoscope blade alters your view. See the anatomy in your mind's eye. Practice intubation at every available opportunity. Rereading this text after such practice will improve your comprehension and retention.

While intubation is a skill that requires practice to master, *anyone can intubate.*

1

Anatomy

T o intubate, you have to manipulate the anatomy to see the best view of the larynx. This is very difficult to do if you don't know how all the structures tie together. Knowledge of normal anatomy lets you identify the landmarks, even when faced with abnormal anatomy.

When you intubate, you place the endotracheal tube between the vocal cords and through a complex structure known as the larynx. The larynx is nothing more than a sophisticated valve with a variety of functions. We breathe through our larynx. It protects our airway from aspiration, the inhalation of foreign material. Its regulation of lung pressures generates the force required to cough. The larynx vibrates the air column to alter pitch and loudness when we speak. It can do these things because of its unique structure.

To feel your own larynx, place your hand on the front of your neck. Identify the firm, roughly cylindrical shape in the midline. Your Adam's apple is part of your larynx (Fig. 1-1, 1-2).

The larynx sits on top of the trachea opposite the fourth, fifth, and sixth cervical vertebrae in the adult. It's a boxlike structure composed of nine cartilages connected by ligaments and moved by nine muscles (Fig. 1-3, 1-4). Far from a static structure, these three single and three paired cartilages pivot and swing in relationship to each other. The connections between the cartilages are true joints with a built in range of motion. Movement of the surrounding tissues shifts the cartilages as well.

Single Cartilages

The single cartilages form the basic structure of the larynx and provide us with our major external landmarks.

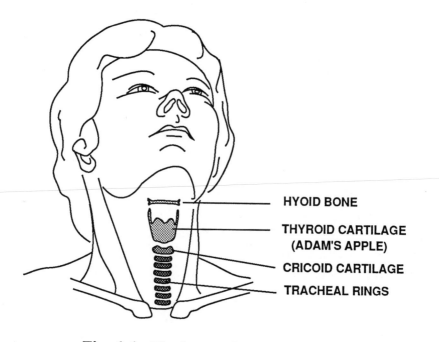

HYOID BONE

THYROID CARTILAGE (ADAM'S APPLE)

CRICOID CARTILAGE

TRACHEAL RINGS

Fig. 1-1. The larynx from the front.

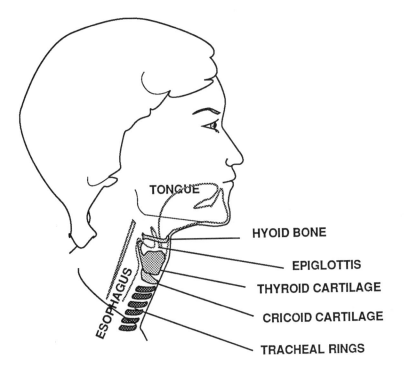

Fig. 1-2. Profile of the larynx.

The **cricoid ring** is signet shaped, with the broad aspect posterior. It sits on top of the first tracheal ring. To easily feel this cartilage, place your fingers on the trachea in the sternal notch and slide them upward. You'll feel a firm, incompressible, ring shaped structure about three to four fingers breadth above the notch. This nondistensible ring is the smallest diameter in the child's airway. Two cricothyroid joints connect the ring anteriorly to the thyroid cartilage, allowing the two to move both independently and as a unit.

The **thyroid cartilage** consists of two quadrangular plates fused anteriorly in the midline. You also know this cartilage as the Adam's apple. Feel this cartilage as a firm projection in the midline of the neck just superior to the cricoid ring. There is a notch on its top edge.

The **epiglottis** is a curved, leaf shaped structure whose upper,

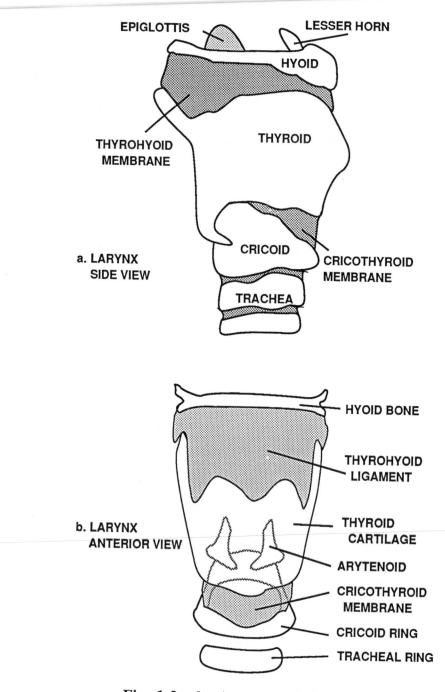

Fig. 1-3a, b. Anatomy of the larynx.

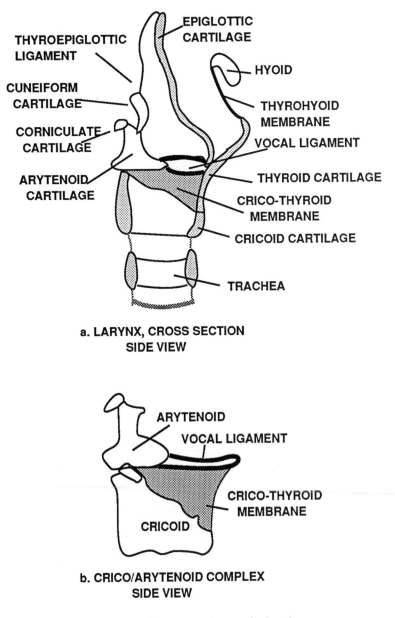

a. LARYNX, CROSS SECTION
SIDE VIEW

b. CRICO/ARYTENOID COMPLEX
SIDE VIEW

Fig. 1-4a, b. Cross-section of the larynx.

rounded edge projects into the pharynx. The stalk of the leaf connects anteriorly to the inside of the thyroid lamina at its midpoint. It also connects to the hyoid bone and to the base of the tongue. You can't feel the epiglottis externally, but it's a major visual landmark in the pharynx when you intubate.

Paired Cartilages

The most important paired cartilages are the **arytenoids**. These are irregular pyramids mounted on top of the posterior aspect of the cricoid cartilage. The signet flange on the ring separates them from each other. The arytenoids are important visual landmarks for intubation. You must be able to recognize their shape. The arytenoids pivot in all planes on the cricoid ring. Each vocal cord projects forward from the sharp anterior vocal process. Movement of the arytenoids tenses, relaxes, and swings the vocal cords from side to side. This lets us phonate, breath, cough, and swallow without aspirating.

The cone shaped **corniculates** attach to the apex of the arytenoids and the elongated **cuneiforms** attach to the posterior arytenoids. They're important to us only because they add bulk and shape to the arytenoid outline.

Tying It All Together: Membranes and Muscles

Several ligaments and two membranes connect the laryngeal cartilages. The most important membrane is the cricoid membrane, which runs from the arytenoids to the thyroid cartilage. The upper free edge of this membrane is the vocal cord.

Normally, the cords are pale and pearly white. Their attachment to the cricoid ring both directly and indirectly explains the success of cricoid pressure. As you'll see, we use downward pressure on the cricoid ring to help bring the vocal cords into view when they are hidden behind the tongue. Pushing on the cricoid pushes the cords.

Structurally, the anterior two thirds is membranous and the posterior one third is cartilaginous. The cartilaginous skeleton allows the vocal cords to close the larynx more effectively if the need arises. It may prevent you from placing an endotracheal tube between closed cords. Forcing a tube through the cords with excessive pressure can actually dislocate an arytenoid and cause permanent hoarseness.

A second membrane, the quadrangular membrane, runs anteriorly from the lateral border of the arytenoids. The upper edge forms the aryepiglottic fold. The lower edge forms the vestibular fold or false vocal cord. The false cords thus lie above the true vocal cords and help close the glottis.

The entire larynx falls on inspiration and rises on expiration. It also rises on coughing, straining, and swallowing. This makes sense. A lower larynx opens the airway while a higher one places the epiglottis and the tongue in better position to close it. Place your hand on your larynx and you can feel the movements.

When at rest, the vocal cords lie partially separated, or abducted. During forceful inspiration or hyperventilation, the cords open widely producing a lozenge shaped opening (Fig. 1-5). This minimizes resistance to breathing. Hyperventilation also makes it easier for us to pass an endotracheal tube in an awake patient.

To produce a high pitched voice, or in response to tracheobronchial irritation, the interarytenoid muscles pinch the cords together, or adduct them.

Injury to the recurrent laryngeal nerve produces vocal cord paralysis on the affected side. A paralyzed cord lies halfway between fully closed and fully open, the cadaveric position. The recurrent laryngeal nerve carries fibers which both separate and approximate the cords. It's easier to damage the more superficial separating fibers. Surgery or trauma sometimes bruises or cuts these fibers. Airway obstruction can occur if the vocal cord dysfunction occurs on both sides because the undamaged approximating fibers pull the cords together.

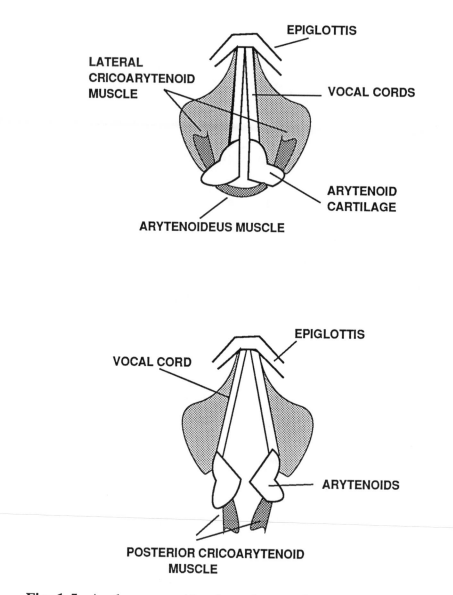

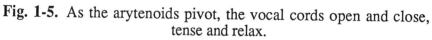

Fig. 1-5. As the arytenoids pivot, the vocal cords open and close, tense and relax.

Closure of the larynx occurs by three mechanisms:

1. closure of the vocal cords

2. closure of the false cords

3. mounding of the paraglottic tissues (lower epiglottis, paraglottic fat, base of tongue) by elevation of the larynx.

The larynx depends so strongly on muscle control that the loss of muscle tone can cause airway obstruction. Soft tissue, including the tongue, falls into the airway and can block the opening. Muscle relaxation narrows the gap between the cords but does not alter gas flow through the larynx. The resultant Bernoulli effect sucks the cords together and produces a high pitched, noisy sound with respiration. This sound, known as stridor, is characteristic of airway obstruction. Obstruction can occur regardless of whether loss of muscle tone comes from unconsciousness, muscle relaxant drugs, or cardiac arrest.

By contrast, light anesthesia, excessive secretions, or aspiration stimulate the airway and activate the defense reflexes. Forceful cord closure and elevation of the larynx seal the airway. Laryngospasm, or spasmotic closure of the vocal cords, is the most severe form of airway closure. Airway obstruction from laryngospasm can totally prevent ventilation. It can physically prevent the passage of an endotracheal tube. You have experienced laryngospasm when you accidentally tried to aspirate water or a pea at dinner. Laryngospasm produced the choking sensation and the loud, stridorous noises you made when you finally succeeded in taking a breath. Carried to extreme your laryngeal protective reflexes prevent air exchange.

Let's turn to the actual appearance of the larynx. Although covered by mucous membrane, you can still see the basic, underlying skeletal shapes. Memorize the view from the top. Look for this view every time you intubate (Fig. 1-6). Try to picture how the underlying skeleton will move when you pull or push on the membrane draped over the top. Knowing the relationships of the structures will let you find the gap between the cords, even if you only see some of the land-marks. Understanding the anatomy puts you in control.

FRONT OF THE PATIENT

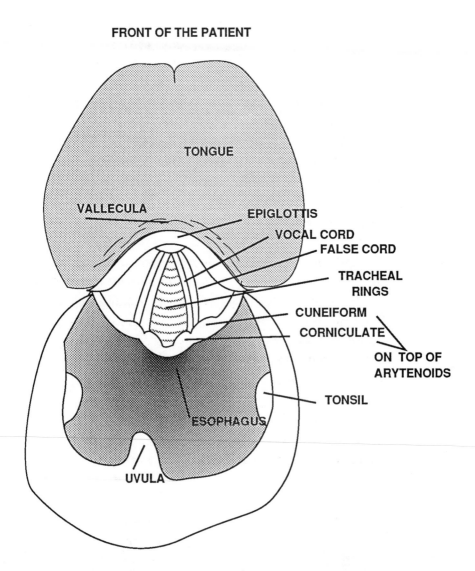

Fig. 1-6. View of the larynx from the top. Front of the patient is at the top of the page.

2

Preintubation Evaluation — Predicting the Difficult Airway

A simple medical history and physical exam will often alert you to potential problems with intubation and airway management. Such forwarning allows you to alter your technique and your equipment from the start. In the elective situation this is no problem.

The emergency situation is more difficult because you won't have the luxury of a prolonged evaluation and leisurely analysis. Fortunately, you can easily spot many of the warning signs of a difficult airway. Additionally, medical care providers at scenes of emergencies can tell you important information if you know what to ask. This rapid analysis lets you rationally choose endotracheal tube size, type and size of laryngoscope blade, and technique.

Medical History

Operations in and around the airway can produce distortion by either changing or removing normal anatomical landmarks. Recent surgery, trauma, tumor, and infection often produce edema or hematoma formation. These not only distort the landmarks but can cause airway obstruction. Nasal fractures often deviate the septum, causing a problem with nasal intubation. Past surgery or irradiation of the neck create scar tissue. This limits the range of motion of the larynx, fixing it in position. It can also limit the range of motion of the head and neck. Anything that alters anatomy or limits motion of the larynx or neck makes difficult intubation more likely.

Physical Signs

Short muscular neck — The larynx on these patients is often higher in the neck, opposite the fourth cervical vertebrae and higher. This makes it harder for the laryngoscope to push the tongue and epiglottis forward. Downward pressure on the vallecula often folds the epiglottis down, hiding the cords. This makes curved blades more difficult to use in these patients. The patient's teeth can be an added disadvantage because teeth limit your ability to maneuver the blade. These patients often require a straight blade and cricoid pressure for intubation.

Receding Chin — Patients with receding chins have hypoplastic or poorly developed mandibles. Again, there is less room to displace the tongue and epiglottis forward. Identify these patients by looking at their profile and noting the chin line. Spot them also by measuring the distance from the inside of the mandible to the hyoid bone with your fingertips. This distance is normally at least three fingers breadths in the adult (Fig. 2-1). Less than three is an indication that you may have difficulty. Two or less almost assures it. Have these patients extend their necks. A distance from the lower border of the mandible to the thyroid notch of less than 6 cm alerts you to potential problems.

Patients with receding chins and those with short necks have a so-called "anterior larynx." Their larynx isn't more anterior in their

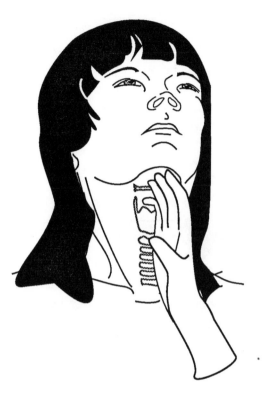

Fig. 2-1. Measuring the distance from the mentum of the chin to the hyoid bone — 3 fingers breadth in the adult.

neck when seen in profile. But when you try to view their larynx with the laryngoscope, the entire structure lies anterior to your field of view (Fig. 2-2). Since the larynx is higher in the neck, there is less room to displace the other structures forward to clear the path to the larynx. The larynx can be very hard to see. Sometimes you only see the arytenoids. At other times you can see no landmarks at all. Straight blades and cricoid pressure should come to mind when you spot the signs.

    Overbite — The presence of an overbite (the protrusion of the incisor teeth due to relative overgrowth of the premaxilla) hampers intubation. There is less room to maneuver your blade. The upper teeth

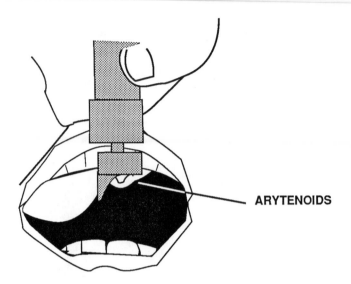

ARYTENOIDS

Fig. 2-2. The view seen with an anterior larynx. Here you can see the arytenoids. Often you see no landmarks.

simply get in the way. In these patients it is especially important to lift the mandible and extend the head as much as possible. This prevents using the teeth as a fulcrum.

Limited Mobility of the Mandible — Opening the mouth requires two movements: opening the hinge joint on a vertical axis and then sliding the angle of the jaw forward. Check both since arthritis, scar tissue, and spasm of the masseter muscle can impair either movement. First check the patient's ability to open the mouth widely (Fig. 2-3). Normally adults can open the mouth at least three cm or about three finger breadths. When a patient can't open that broadly, it impairs your ability to maneuver and to see. You may not be able to insert your blade at all.

Second, check the ability to displace the mandible. Have the patient push his lower jaw forward to place his lower teeth in front of his upper teeth (Fig 2-4). If he or she can't, you might not be able to pull the mandible forward far enough to see the larynx. Patients with temporomandibular joint arthritis frequently lose the forward glide of their jaw before they lose their ability to open their mouths.

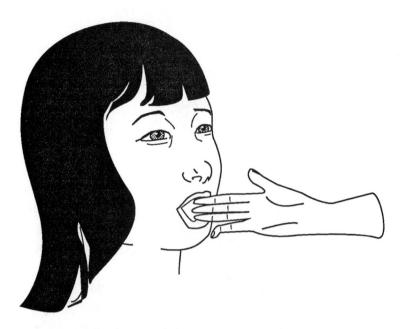

Fig. 2-3. Can the patient open his or her mouth wide enough for 3 fingers?

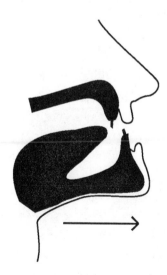

Fig. 2-4. Have the patients place their lower teeth outside their upper teeth to check for the ability of their jaw to glide forward.

Oral Cavity — There are a number of things to check here. First, look at the condition of the teeth. Notice teeth that are loose, chipped, or missing before you start. Look at the relative size of the tongue in relation to the rest of the mouth. Young children have relatively large tongues. Sometimes, patients with oral tumors or trauma have a swollen or enlarged tongue. High arched palates with narrow mouths make passage of the tube difficult because the blade itself takes up so much room.

Finally, have the erect patient open his mouth as widely as possible and look at the posterior pharynx. You can use Mallampati's signs and classification to identify patients at risk for difficult intubation (Fig. 2-5). Visibility of intraoral structures correlates with ease of viewing with a laryngoscope. Patients in categories I and II are low risk. Patients in category III and IV are at high risk for problems.

Flexion and extension of the Neck — Have the patient touch his chin to his chest (normal 45°) and to both shoulders in turn (normal 40°). Then have the patient extend his head back as far as possible (normal 55°). Normal range of motion decreases about 20% by 70 years of age. Limited range of motion impairs your ability to bring the axes into alignment.

External larynx — Look at the trachea and the external laryngeal structures. Are they midline in the neck or deviated to one side? Tumor, trauma, hematoma, and scar tissue can deviate the trachea. Movement of the larynx from the midline makes indentification of landmarks and alignment of axes more difficult. Place your hand over the larynx and gently move it from side to side. A larynx fixed to the midline by tumor or scar is often hard to lift with the laryngoscope. It looks anterior and is often very hard to see (Fig. 2-6).

Vocal cords — Indirect exam of the vocal cords entails listening to the voice. The presence of hoarseness can mean edema, tumor, paralysis, or arthritis. All of the above imply the need for a smaller than average endotracheal tube. I try to place the largest tube possible for the patient — to minimize the need for excessive cuff inflation, to assist suctioning, and to minimize airway resistance. However, I will

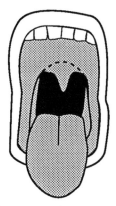

Class I: soft palate, uvula,
fauces, pillars visible

No difficulty

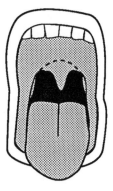

Class II: soft palate, uvula,
fauces visible

No difficulty

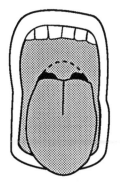

Class III: soft palate, base
of uvula visible

Moderate difficulty

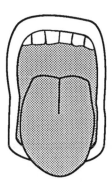

Class IV: hard palate
only visible

Severe difficulty

Fig. 2-5. Mallampati Signs as indicators of difficulty of intubation.
(Adapted from Mallampati and Samsoon and Young)

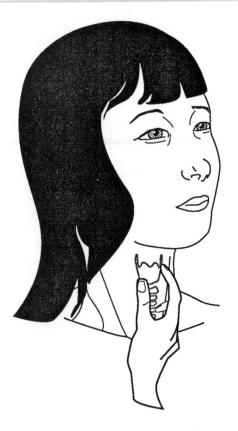

Fig. 2-6. Gently move the larynx from side to side to check for masses and immobility.

often start with a smaller tube if I expect a smaller opening. This is especially true in emergencies when I don't want to risk inability to pass the tube on the first try.

You can examine the vocal cords with an indirect laryngoscopy mirror before intubation if there is any question of possible obstruction. Special, soft tissue X-rays and other studies may also be helpful in the non-emergent situation.

Nose — Checking the nose is important if you plan a nasal intubation. Ask the patient if he has everbroken his nose. Is the septum deviated? Check to see if he can breath equally out both sides or if one side is more patent. Is there a history of nose bleeds or sinusitis, which may predispose the patient to complications from a nasal intubation?

Remember that patients who are potentially difficult to intubate may also be difficult to ventilate if given a general anesthetic. If you have any doubt about your ability to ventilate the patient, you should place the tube with the patient awake.

In the emergency situation you will not have time to perform a detailed physical exam or take an involved history. However, you can learn many things by just looking at the patient and asking a few questions as you prepare your equipment. A few well-spent minutes before you start often prevents a difficult and prolonged intubation attempt.

Let's imagine that you've been called to intubate a patient that you don't know. Ask the following questions while you prepare to intubate.

1. Why does this patient need intubation? The answer to this question will let you know how quickly you need to proceed. Cardiac arrest victims and patients dying from lack of oxygen require fast action. Progressive respiratory failure in an asthmatic who is tiring, but still ventilating, allows more time for analysis.

2. Is someone ventilating this patient? Regardless of the reason for intubation, your first duty in the room is to be sure that the patient is being ventilated and oxygenated. *Ventilation takes priority over everything else.* If you are the only one capable of ventilating the patient, do so. Have an assistant prepare your equipment.

3. What important medical problems does this patient have? Knowing that an awake patient with respiratory failure also has unstable angina is important if you are to minimize hypertension and stress during intubation. Knowing that a patient suffers from AIDS or hepatitis is important to know to protect yourself during the intubation. Nasal

intubations are relatively contraindicated in immunosuppressed patients and those with diabetes because of the risk of sinusitus.

4. Is this patient anticoagulated? Intubation techniques in the anticoagulated patient must be especially gentle to prevent bleeding into the airway. Additionally, you should not perform a nasal intubation in an anticoagulated patient due to the risk of nose bleed.

5. Is there any problem with the airway? When I encounter a history of surgery, trauma, tumor, radiation or infection of the airway I reach for a straight, rather than a curved, blade and for a smaller, rather than a larger, tube.

During this exchange you are quickly choosing what you feel is the appropriate laryngoscope blade and tube. You are checking the cuff on the tube for leaks and inserting a stylet. And you are asking for suction — with a yankauer suction tip if possible. Suction is often a low priority item for the resuscitation team. It is a high priority item for you because you need to see the larynx and you need to clear the airway.

A quick look at the patient identifies such signs as a receding chin, an overbite, facial trauma, a deviated trachea, and a short, thick neck. Ventilating the patient before the intubation identifies problems with neck and jaw mobility. It took less than the 2-4 minutes you needed to prepare your equipment to do a simple evaluation of the patient's airway.

Equipment

T o intubate you need an endotracheal tube, and the ability to identify the larynx, suction the airway, and ventilate the patient. Most emergency settings in the United States have specialized equipment readily available. Optimally, you should have the following list of supplies.

Equipment you need for intubation includes:

- laryngoscope handle with functioning batteries

- laryngoscope blade with functioning light bulb, both straight and curved if possible

- proper sizes of endotracheal tubes

- suction apparatus, with yankauer and flexible catheters

- syringe for inflating endotracheal tube cuff

- stylet

Equipment you should have for airway management includes:

- mask and bag ventilating apparatus

- oral airway

- nasal airway

- oxygen supply

- Magill forceps

- means of securing tube, such as tape

- stethoscope for checking proper tube placement

We'll discuss the use of all the equipment later. Now let's concentrate on checking the equipment for functionality.

Checking Your Laryngoscope

First check your laryngoscope blade and handle. To attach the blade to the handle notice that the handle has a post on top — inside of a square depression. The blade has a matching hook shaped flange. Hold the handle in your left hand and the blade in your right so the flange hooks over the post and seats into the depression (Fig. 3-1a). Push the blade forward until you feel it snap into place (Fig. 3-1b). The blade will be at an angle to the handle. The fit should be snug so the blade does not fall off the handle when in the off position.

To turn the laryngoscope on, pull the blade into a right angle with the handle (Fig. 3-1c). Again you should feel a snap as it locks. The light should turn on. If it doesn't, tighten the light bulb connection. If the bulb still fails to light, change the batteries and/or the bulb and try again. Finally, remove the blade and check the contact points between the blade and the handle. Occasionally you must clean the contacts just as you clean the contacts on a battery. Use an alcohol swab, an eraser, or an emory board. You should periodically check the intubation equipment

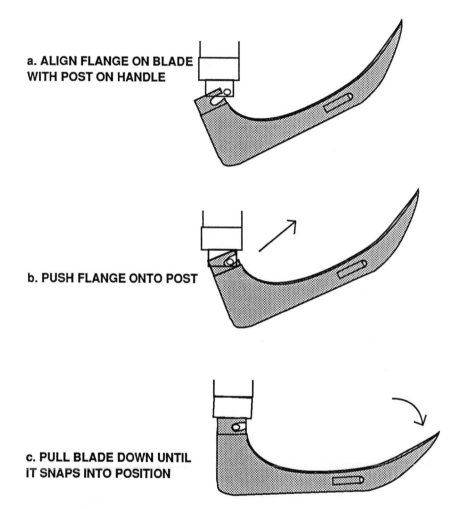

a. ALIGN FLANGE ON BLADE
WITH POST ON HANDLE

b. PUSH FLANGE ONTO POST

c. PULL BLADE DOWN UNTIL
IT SNAPS INTO POSITION

Fig. 3-1. Placing the blade on your laryngoscope.

before you need it. Trouble shooting in the middle of an emergency is inappropriate.

If you haven't done so, look at the differences between a curved and a straight blade. There are many variations of straight and curved blades. The most common ones in use are the curved MacIntosh blades and the straight Miller blades (Fig. 3-2, 3-3).

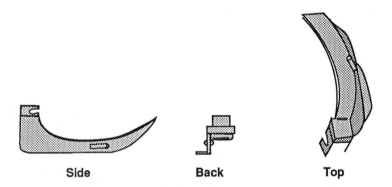

Side   Back   Top

Fig. 3-2. Macintosh Blade. Notice the position of the light bulb, the broad, flat blade width, the tall flange for positioning the tongue, and the overall curved shape.

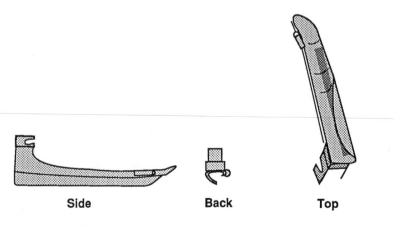

Side   Back   Top

Fig. 3-3. Miller Blade. Notice the position of light bulb, the narrow blade width, the curved channel in center, and the overall straight shape.

Checking Your Endotracheal Tube

Next, check the endotracheal tube cuff (Fig. 3-4). Attach your syringe, usually a ten cc syringe, to the pilot balloon and distend the cuff with air. Detach the syringe and check to see if the cuff leaks — as shown by the loss of air. Leaks can occur in either the cuff or in the balloon assembly. By keeping the tube inside the sterile wrapper you can squeeze the cuff without contaminating it.

You should be aware that endotracheal tube cuffs may break during intubation if they snag on the teeth, etc. Hence tubes, which initially tested fine, may leak after the intubation.

I recommend discarding any tube which leaks. However, there are times when changing a leaking tube in an intubated patient may be difficult. For example, a cuff leak which develops in the middle of head and neck surgery can be hard to treat. You lack easy access to the patient's airway. A long term ventilator patient in the intensive care unit is another example. Occasionally these patients won't tolerate even limited interruption in ventilation without becoming cyanotic. Change the tube if you can.

If you can't, first check the pilot tube. Inflate the cuff until the leak stops and keep the pilot balloon sealed with a closed stopcock or

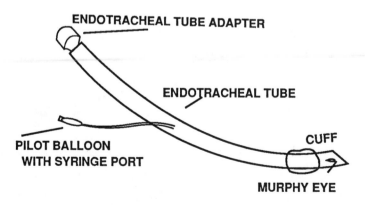

Fig. 3-4. Parts of an endotracheal tube.

syringe. If the cuff retains air with the pilot tube plugged, then the pilot tube is probably leaking. To keep the cuff inflated use a closed stopcock, a syringe with the plunger firmly taped, or a clamp on the pilot tube itself. I usually avoid clamping the pilot tube itself. This permanently seals the balloon and prevents you from adding any more air in the future.

When the cuff itself leaks, you can temporarily pack the posterior pharynx around the tube with gauze. This helps prevent aspiration and plugs the leak. *Always remember to remove the pack* when you remove or change the tube. Packs left in the pharynx cause potentially fatal airway obstruction. Please view these tricks as temporary measures and not long term solutions.

Placing Your Stylet

Placing your stylet inside the tube comes next (Fig. 3-5). You can intubate without a stylet and you should practice doing so. I always use one in emergency situations. Failure to intubate rapidly here can lead to aspiration and lack of oxygen. Lubricate the stylet before you insert it. You can use a local anesthetic or lubricating gel, or plain water. Slide

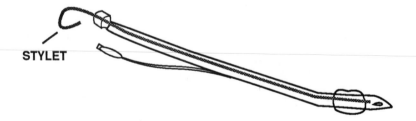

STYLET

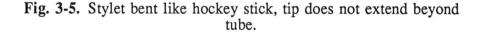

Fig. 3-5. Stylet bent like hockey stick, tip does not extend beyond tube.

the stylet into the tube. Make sure that the stylet does not extend beyond the tip of the tube because the stylet can gouge the trachea in this position. Bend the tip of the endotracheal tube slightly so the tube looks like a hockey stick. This helps you if the patient has an anterior larynx. Make sure that you can still pull the bent stylet out easily. Lubricating gel can occasionally dry out and get sticky. If the stylet has been in the tube a while make sure it's not stuck before you intubate. Nothing is more embarrassing than successfully intubating a patient only to be unable to take the stylet out of the tube.

Final Details

Finally, check that you have suction ready. Also make sure you have the connecting tubing, suction catheters, extension cords, and the power to go with it.

Have the means to ventilate the patient present. Appropriately sized masks, oral and nasal airways (Fig. 3-6), and oxygen should be available. Magill forceps are often useful if you need to do a nasal intubation.

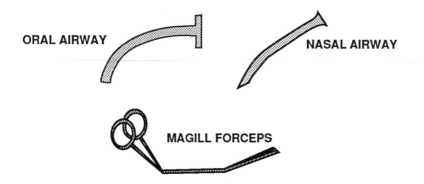

ORAL AIRWAY

NASAL AIRWAY

MAGILL FORCEPS

Fig. 3-6. Airway equipment to have present during an intubation.

What To Do When
You Don't Have Optimal Equipment

The reason I originally referred to the list of suggested equipment as optimal is simple. On occasion you may have to intubate a patient without all of the equipment available. Be flexible and let your knowledge of the anatomy and of what you need to accomplish be your guide.

You can intubate a patient without a functioning laryngoscope in several ways. First, use your unlighted laryngoscope or some other similarly shaped instrument such as a bent spoon or oral speculum to lift the jaw. Have an assistant hold a flashlight up to the outside of the larynx. This illuminates the larynx through the skin and the vocal cords light up. Once you can see them you can pass your tube. You can also intubate by feel. Place the fingers of your left hand inside the patient's mouth until your index and middle fingers straddle the larynx. Pass the endotracheal tube with your right hand, using your left hand to direct it between the vocal cords.

If you don't have a ventilation bag use mouth-to-mouth or mouth-to-tube ventilation.

Active suction is wonderful. Improvise it if you don't have it. Quickly turn the patient on his or her side to clear the airway with gauze or other tissue. Use a syringe bulb or a syringe attached to some IV extension tubing.

Have someone place an ear to the chest and listen for breath sounds if you don't have a stethoscope.

Always open your mind to alternatives. Flexibility saves patient's lives.

4

Oral Intubation
of the Adult Patient

Many of you have already intubated an intubation mannequin and therefore are familiar with the basic technique. However, intubating the dummy differs from intubating the typical patient. You should recognize these differences before you approach your first patient.

The Dummy vs. the Real Thing

The dummy's plastic face is very stiff and noncompliant. You've probably noticed that the mouth already lies fully open and is difficult to open further. In contrast, you must open the patient's mouth, and do so without getting in the way of your laryngoscope. Being soft and very compliant, the human cheek will hang limply, obstructing the view.

   The dummy's head is so light that it takes little effort to lift the entire mannequin off the table. Often instructors have to hold the mannequin on the table to help the trainee out. In contrast, the average adult head weighs about 5 lbs. The added weight makes balancing the head on the blade and lifting the head into the proper alignment technically more difficult. Holding the head in proper position, especially through a long and difficult intubation, is very tiring.

You can often see the dummy's larynx even without the laryngoscope lit because the pale plastic reflects light so well. This isn't the case in humans. The mucous membranes are dark. The larynx, deep in the hole, lies in shadow. Placing the laryngoscope light correctly and then interpreting the view is easier if you know what the real larynx looks like.

The dummy's tongue is fairly firm, difficult to shift from side to side. However, it will remain out of the way of your blade. Your patient's tongue will be a soft, very slippery mound of flesh. It will invariably be in the worst position to block your view if you fail to control it.

Psychology is the final difference. You know that you cannot hurt the dummy even if you fail completely. Every beginner fears his or her first patient intubation. Even if you can intubate the dummy with your eyes closed I guarantee that your first few intubations will be frightening. This is normal. You worry about failure because you doubt your ability to succeed. You are fearful of what will happen if you fail. However, if you approach the patient with gentle, purposeful movements, and ventilate the patient between attempts, your likelihood of hurting the patient is low. Panic hurts patients. Apprehension does not. Use your apprehension as a tool to heighten your awareness and to promote caution. If you believe you can intubate, you will.

Intubating the Adult

To orally intubate you need to bring the path from the incisor teeth to the larynx into a straight line. This path has three axes (Fig. 4-1):

1. axis of the cavity of the mouth (oral axis)

2. axis of the cavity of the pharynx (pharyngeal axis)

3. axis of the larynx and trachea (laryngeal axis)

The angle of the axis of the mouth to the larynx is 90°. That of the pharynx to the trachea is obtuse. Aligning them is merely a matter of applied mechanics. You make this alignment by moving the patient's head and neck and then using the laryngoscope blade to make the final adjustment. Other techniques can be used if you should not move the patient's head, such as in cervical trauma and some facial fractures. We'll discuss these situations in chapter 8. Here we discuss the basic intubation technique assuming optimal conditions.

Place the patient's head at the level of your xyphoid, the lower tip of your breast bone for the best mechanical advantage. You can, however, intubate in any position.

The act of intubation alternates hands. One hand positions the patient for the next action by the other hand. With practice, coordinating the alternating hand movements becomes natural.

Raise the patient's head about 10 cm (4 inches) off the bed by placing a folded sheet or other object under their head. Leave the shoulders

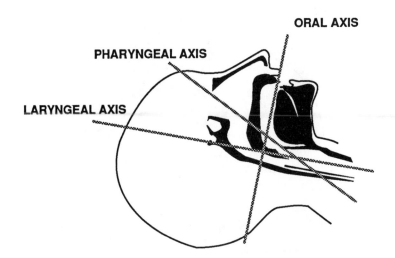

Fig. 4-1. The three axes with the head in neutral position.

on the bed (Fig. 4-2). This aligns the pharyngeal and laryngeal axes. The cervical spine is now straight and the patient is in the so-called "sniffing position." Picture how someone out of breath holds her head: forward and tilted slightly back. We automatically straighten the airway to minimize resistance when we want to move a lot of air easily.

Tilt the head into extension with your right hand. This brings all the axes into alignment (Fig. 4-3). Hold it there momentarily either by using your upper chest or your left hand to anchor it (Fig. 4-4a, b). Don't stick your fingers into the patient's eyes as you do this! Anchoring the head frees your right hand. Open the mouth with your right hand by placing your thumb on the lower jaw and your middle finger on the upper jaw (Fig. 4-5a, b). The position is similar to snapping your fingers. By using a pushing rather than a spreading motion, you can open the mouth wider and more forcefully. Make sure that you place your fingers as far to the right side of the mouth as you can. This keeps your fingers out of the way of the blade.

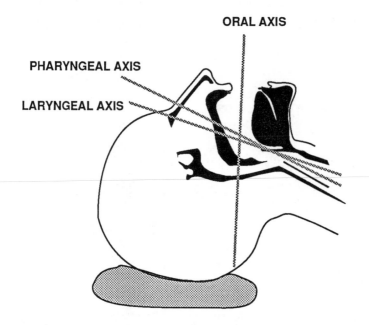

ORAL AXIS

PHARYNGEAL AXIS

LARYNGEAL AXIS

Fig. 4-2. The three axes with the head in the "sniffing" position.

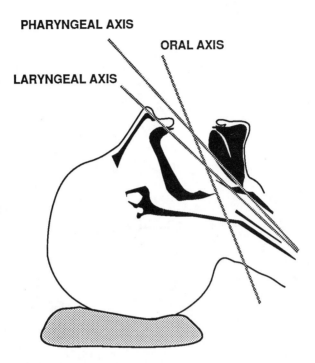

PHARYNGEAL AXIS

ORAL AXIS

LARYNGEAL AXIS

Fig. 4-3. The three axes after extending the head.

Your right hand now does double duty. It holds the mouth open as wide as it can. By pulling toward you it also holds the head in extension. You can now step back from the head and use your left hand to pick up and insert the blade (Fig. 4-6).

Insertion of the blade should be delicate and deliberate. Hold the handle in your left hand, blade down, pointing away from you (Fig. 4-7). Don't clench your fist because this decreases control and causes early fatigue. Because my hands are small, I place my hand lower down on the handle. I rest my fifth finger on the blade and wrap my hand around the handle. This puts the heel of my hand on the junction between blade and handle and allows me to fine tune the angle of the blade. Notice how easily you can change the angle of the blade by tilting your wrist (Fig. 4-7a, b).

With the mouth open, insert the blade between the teeth, slightly to

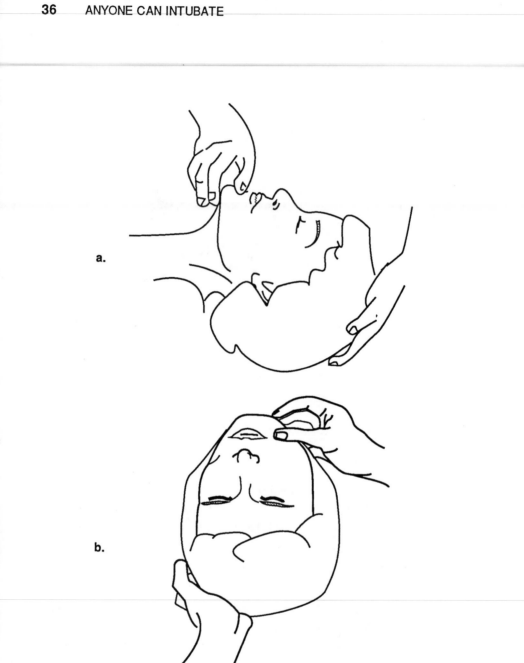

a.

b.

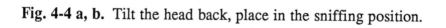

Fig. 4-4 a, b. Tilt the head back, place in the sniffing position.

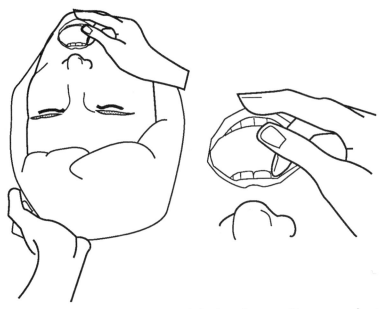

Fig. 4-5. Open the mouth with your right hand, your fingers as far to the right of the mouth as possible. Notice the positioning of the fingers.

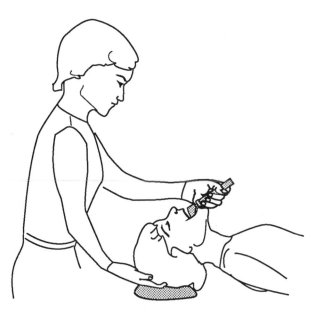

Fig. 4-6. Keep your back and your left arm straight to optimize mechanical advantage.

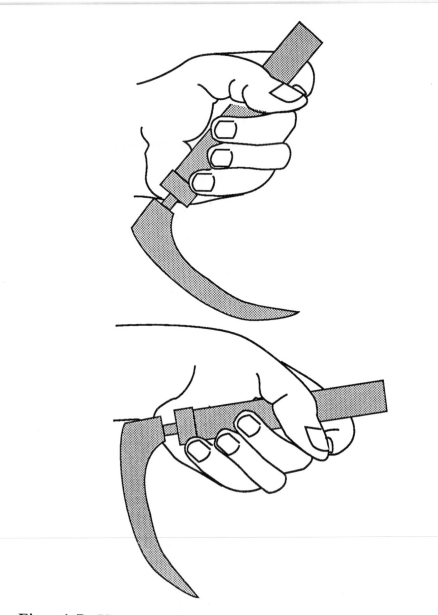

Fig. 4-7. You can easily change the angle of the blade by rotating your wrist.

the right of the tongue (Fig. 4-8a, b). Don't push on the teeth as you do so. Also avoid catching the lips between the blade and the teeth. I use my right index finger to sweep the lips out of the way of the blade as I insert it.

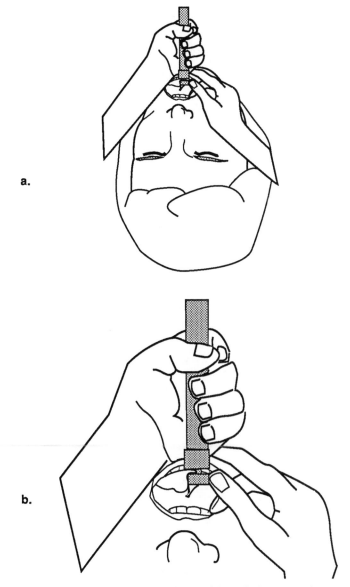

Fig. 4-8. Insert the blade on the right side of the mouth, not in the middle of the tongue.

Slowly advance the blade with your left hand until you see the tip of the epiglottis, your first important landmark. Simultaneously sweep the tongue to the left as you advance (Fig. 4-9a, b). This leaves your

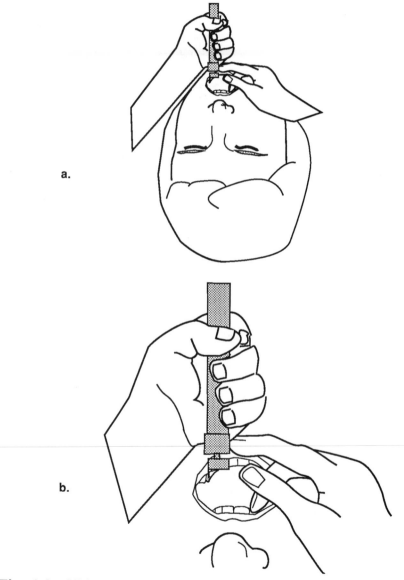

a.

b.

Fig. 4-9. Slide the blade to the left, pushing the tongue out of the way. Lift upward on the lower jaw.

blade in the midline of the mouth with the tongue pushed out of the way. When you lift the jaw upward you have an unobstructed view of the larynx (Fig. 4-10a, b, c). Pressure from the tip of a curved blade in the vallecula pulls the epiglottis forward. Placement of the blade is critical. If you place the blade in the center of the tongue it will mound up and you will see nothing. You must sweep the tongue to the left or you will see nothing.

For optimal mechanical advantage lift upward with the left arm held fairly straight. Lift on a line connecting the patient's head with the intersection of the opposite ceiling and the wall (Fig. 4-11). Keeping your arm straight gives you the strength of your shoulders to lift the head. It prevents you from using the teeth as a fulcrum — dangerous for the teeth. And it allows you to use binocular vision for depth perception. The typical beginners (Fig. 4-12) hunch close to the patient, bend the elbow completely, and place the right eye practically into the patient's mouth. They then can't understand why he or she has no leverage or control. Don't do this.

Back to the intubation. We left you with the head virtually suspended from the blade held in your left hand. This frees your right hand to place the tube. Use a 7-8 for a woman and a 7.5 -8.5 for a man. Size 9-10 tubes are rarely needed. Hold the pre-selected tube in your right hand like a pencil, curve forward. In one smooth motion pass the tube into the larynx through the cords (Fig. 4-13). If the patient is breathing, time the forward thrust for inspiration when the cords open. During expiration, the tube may bounce off the cords into the esophagus. Beginners frequently try to pass the tube down the slot in the blade. The slot is not big enough for this purpose. Instead, pass the tube to the right of the blade, past the right side of the tongue. This is the major reason why the blade has to be as far to the left side of the mouth as possible.

Try to watch the tube pass through the cords into the trachea. Although there may be a blind spot impairing your view at the moment of intubation, you can often see the arytenoids behind the tube after proper placement. Don't relax and pull the blade out without trying to be sure of success with your own eyes. Get into the habit of seeing the

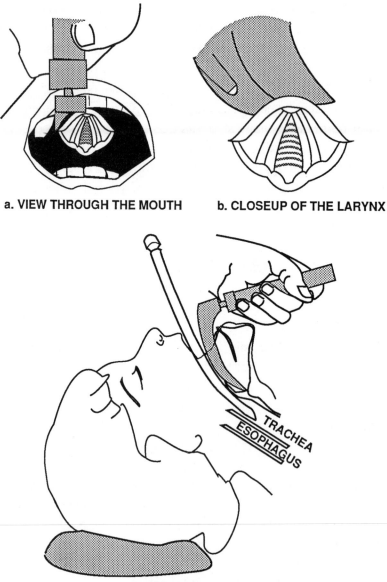

a. VIEW THROUGH THE MOUTH   b. CLOSEUP OF THE LARYNX

TRACHEA
ESOPHAGUS

c. CROSS SECTION OF THE INTUBATION

Fig. 4-10. Visualization of the cords and passing the endotracheal tube.

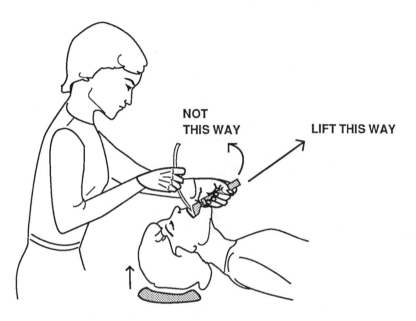

Fig. 4-11. Proper technique for lifting the head.

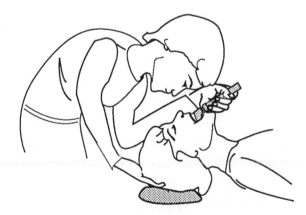

Fig. 4-12. Avoid stooping over the patient and bending your arm. You lose mechanical advantage, binocular vision, and maneuverability.

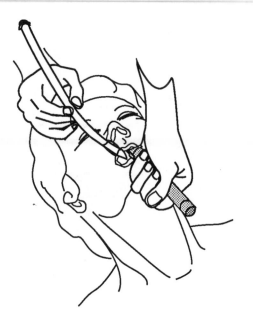

Fig. 4-13. Another view of passing the tube into the larynx.

tube between the cords and you will be less likely to intubate the esophagus.

Stop advancing the tube when you see the cuff completely pass the cords. Carefully hold the tube where it exits the right side of the mouth and remove the blade with your left hand. To inflate the cuff to the minimal sealing pressure, apply constant airway pressure of about 20 mmHg. Then fill the cuff with air until the tracheal leak just disappears. Excessive cuff inflation can damage mucosa by impairing its blood supply.

Before doing anything else, be sure that the tube is in the trachea. Listen for the presence and equality of breath sounds over both lung fields and for the absence of gurgling sounds over the stomach. Never assume that the tube is in the trachea until you have checked it yourself. More details on this later.

Securing the Tube

Next, tape the tube securely. Only your taping stands between the patient and extubation. To start, notice the depth of the tube by looking at the numbers. Remember which number lines up with the front gum line: typically 21 cm for a woman, 22 cm for a man. For a child the depth in centimeters should equal the age in years divided by 2 plus 12. For example a four year old child should have the tube inserted to a depth of 14cm (or 4 divided by 2 plus 12). Tape the tube to the side of the mouth. It usually doesn't matter on which side of the mouth you tape the tube. Most of us tape it on the right side since the tube already exits from that side. There are many acceptable ways of taping the tube. Figures 4-14 and 4-15 show two ways. These methods have several factors in common. First, having the tube in the exact corner of the mouth is more comfortable for the patient. It avoids the patient pushing the tube out with the tongue. It also makes it easier for others to suction the mouth and place oral airways if needed. Second, you don't leave a tape tether. Tape extensions let the tube slide in or out of the mouth, risking either mainstem intubation or extubation. Finally, you avoid taping over the vermillion border or edge of the lip. You can tear this border when you remove the tape, especially in babies and geriatric patients. In addition, tape over the lips gets wet from saliva and loses its grip.

Once the tube is taped, check again that the tube still lies in the trachea.

If you need the tube on the left side of the mouth, then you will have to move the tube. Hold the tube securely with your right hand where it exits the mouth and rest your hand on the cheek. (Fig. 4-16). Holding further out on the tube is unstable and risks extubation if the head moves. Take a tongue blade, or your laryngoscope blade, with your left hand and open the mouth. Push the tongue firmly down. Under direct vision move the tube from the groove on the right side of the tongue to the groove on the left. Don't let the tube overlie the tongue as this allows the patient to "tongue" it out. Hold the tube

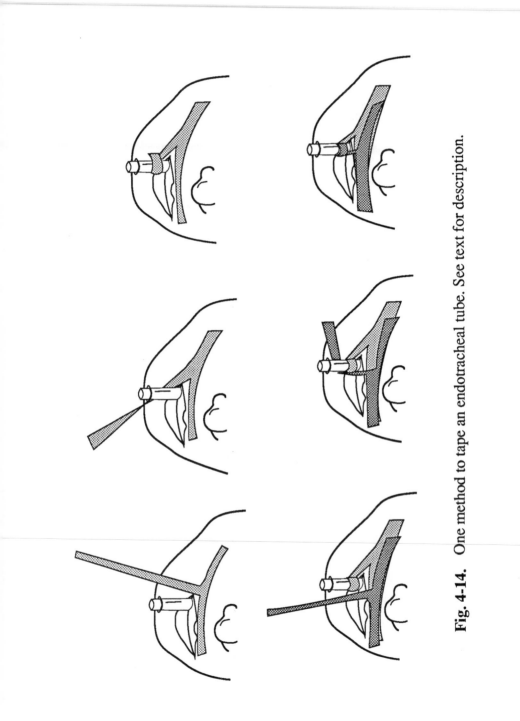

Fig. 4-14.   One method to tape an endotracheal tube. See text for description.

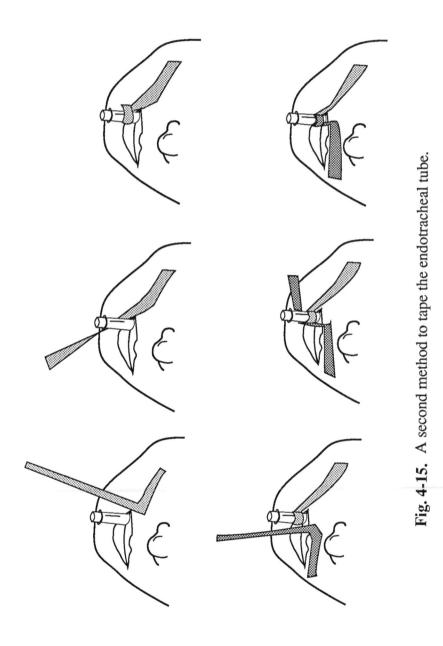

Fig. 4-15. A second method to tape the endotracheal tube.

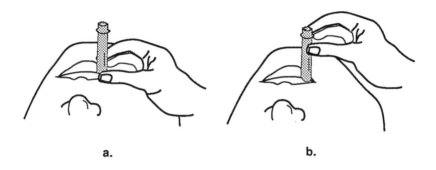

a.   b.

Fig. 4-16. When holding an endotracheal tube, hold it where it exits the mouth as in **a.** Rest your hand against the cheek so that you move as the head moves. Extubation is more likely if you hold the tube as in **b.**

securely with either hand and immediately check that the tube is still in the trachea. I can't emphasize strongly enough that you must verify good breath sounds bilaterally anytime the tube or the patient moves. Extubation and mainstem intubation can occur at any time.

Tape sticks poorly to hair. Taping endotracheal tubes in patients with beards and mustaches requires an alteration in technique. One can use the above methods after applying benzoin to the hair. A more secure method uses an "around the neck" tape as in Fig. 4-17. You can use this method whenever you need greater tube stabilization, for example, during prone positioning or transportation. Don't tape too tightly because your tape might constrict the neck like a tourniquet and cause facial swelling.

Straight vs. Curved Blades

The straight blade, such as the Miller, actually picks up the epiglottis during the intubation. The curved MacIntosh (Mac) blade fits into the vallecula, the dip between the tongue and the epiglottis. While the technique is the same, the effect on the tissues differs between the blades.

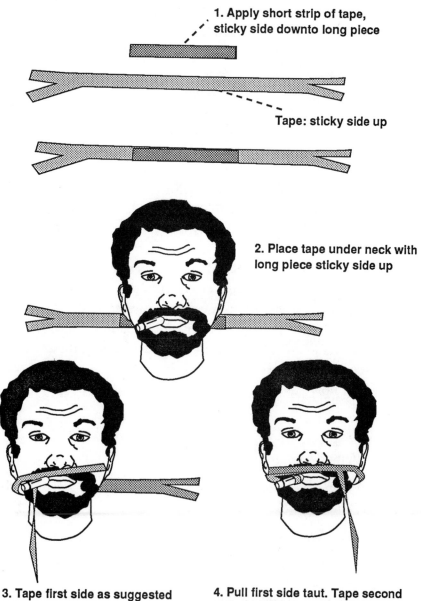

Fig. 4-17. Taping an endotracheal tube with a bearded patient.

The curved blade lifts the epiglottis passively by pulling the tissue folds attached at its base. The straight blade flattens the tongue and actively lifts the epiglottis. See Figures 4-18, 4-19, 4-20 for illustrations of these effects.

You can begin to see that a straight blade might be more helpful in situations where there is little room to displace the tongue and attached tissues forward. Patients with short necks, high larynxes, or obesity frequently need straight blades. Straight blades can also work better in patients with larynxes fixed from scar, trauma, or mass effect. Again, displacement is not as critical. Remember that you can pick up the epiglottis with the Mac or use the Miller in the vallecula if the need arises.

In the average patient, it really doesn't matter which blade you use. Many beginners find the Mac blade easier to use. It's larger flange holds the tongue off to the left and makes it easier to balance the head. It is more forgiving of placement errors. Straight blades often give you a better view but are harder to use. Practice with both blades on the easy patients. That way, when a difficult intubation comes along you control the anatomy rather than letting the anatomy dictate to you. We'll discuss more on these situations later. Look at the pictures and get a feel for how your blade moves the tissues around.

Extubation

Learning to intubate includes learning how and when to safely extubate a patient. Criteria for extubation include:

- recovery of airway reflexes and response to comand
- no hypoxia, hypercarbia, or major acid/base imbalance
- no cardiopulmonary instability
- inspiratory capacity of at least 15 ml/kg
- signs of intact muscle power

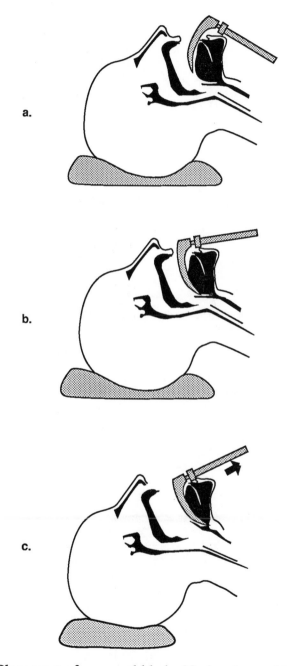

Fig. 4-18. Placement of a curved blade. Notice the position of the tip in the vallecula.

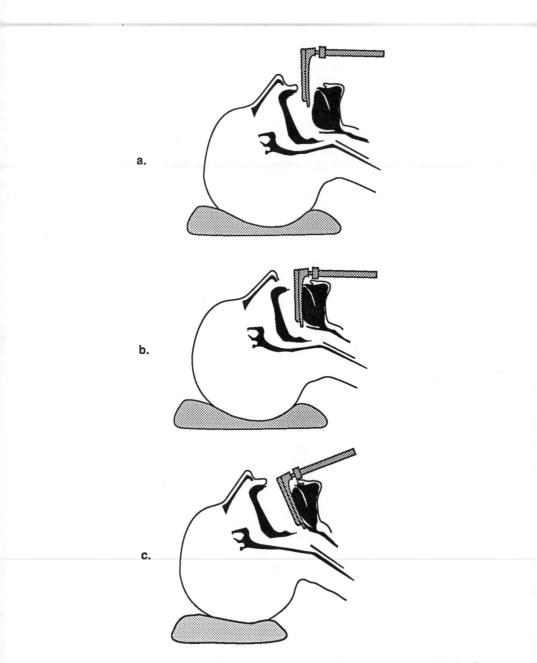

Fig. 4-19. Placement of a straight blade. Notice that the blade flattens the tissue. The tip is on the epiglottis.

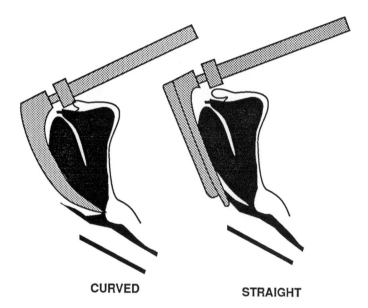

CURVED   **STRAIGHT**

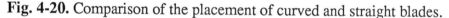

Fig. 4-20. Comparison of the placement of curved and straight blades.

- absence of retraction during spontaneous respiration
- absence of a distended stomach

In other words, you want your patient to be stable, able to breathe without help, and able to protect the airway.

Always suction the pharynx well prior to extubation because oral secretions drain into the trachea when you deflate the cuff. Also suction the endotracheal tube if there are secretions in it. Oxygenate the patient both before and after you suction the tube. Limit the time spent suctioning the tube to less than 10 seconds to prevent hypoxia. Make multiple passes if you have to clear a lot of secretions and oxygenate between each pass.

After you have suctioned and oxygenated the patient, untape the tube. Have the patient take a deep breath, deflate the cuff, and then pull the tube out quickly. The order of steps is important. If the lungs are already inflated then the initial gas flow is outward. Frequently this will blow any secretions sticking to the cuff into the mouth where you can suction them. Squeezing the ventilation bag at the moment of extubation also helps blow secretions out. Deflation of the cuff should immediately preceed extubation for the same reason, to prevent aspiration around the tube.

There is a high risk of laryngospasm and vomiting following extubation. Have suction, oxygen, and the means to reintubate the patient immediately available.

Further Reading

Mallampati SR, Gratt SP, Gugino LD, Desai SP, et. al.: A clinical sign to predict difficult tracheal intubation: a prospective study. *Can. Anaesth. Soc. J.* 1985; 32: 4: 429

Stoelting RK, Miller RD: Airway Management. *Basics of Anesthesia.* Edited by Stoelting RK, Miller RD. New York. Churchill-Livingstone 1984, 153-165

Common Errors
and How To Avoid Them

I nexperienced intubators often make several fairly common errors. Every year new trainees repeat them.

Positioning Errors

Poor head placement is the most common error. Sometimes you can't avoid it, such as during a cardiac arrest with the patient on the floor. Frequently you can optimize position with pillows. Having an assistant stabilize or lift the head, or changing the bed height, are also helpful. These changes are fast, easy to perform, and often forgotten in the heat of battle. They make the intubation easier and therefore less stressful and more likely to succeed.

Keep your left arm and back as straight as possible. Hunching over the patient, a common mistake, makes intubation more difficult because it impairs your mechanical advantage (Fig. 5-1).

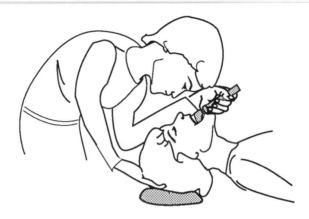

Fig. 5-1. Don't hunch over the patient. Keep your back and left arm as straight as possible.

In the rush to extend the patient's head the intubator will frequently place fingers in the patient's eyes (Fig. 5-2). After all, the orbital ridge is a convenient place to grab and pull. In their preoccupation, they sometimes don't notice themselves doing this.

When opening the mouth, inexperienced fingers grab the middle teeth. This never leaves enough room to pass the blade into the mouth. Place your fingers on the far right. Use the finger positioning shown in Fig. 5-3 and use a pushing rather than a spreading motion.

Left-handed Intubation

Open the mouth as widely as you can. You are far less likely to damage teeth or gums if you give yourself room to maneuver and see.

Most people are right handed. Therefore, many people instinctively reach for the laryngoscope with their right hand. They discover their mistake when they find themselves with their right hand blocking their view and with no way for their left hand to pass a tube over their right. Standard laryngoscopes are held in the non-dominant left hand because this hand merely provides a stable platform. The dominant

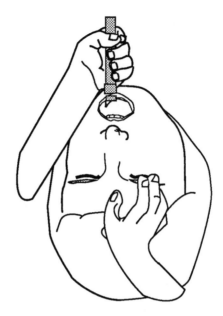

Fig. 5-2. Don't gouge the eyes.

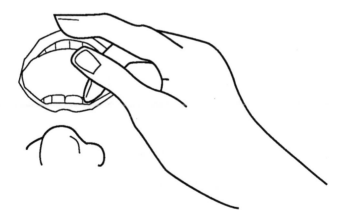

Fig. 5-3. Finger position for opening the mouth.

right hand needs all the coordination and dexterity to manipulate the tube.

Unfortunately, this leaves left handed intubators in an awkward position. As just pointed out, the standard blades are held in the left hand. Reversing them doesn't work. Although the southpaw can purchase a left handed blade, which is a mirror image of the standard blade, I don't recommend this. It is far better for you to train yourself to do it "backwards." Training yourself on left handed tools puts you at a major disadvantage when only right handed tools are available. Most hospitals only stock right handed instruments. It may not be fair, but it's definitely more practical. Most left handed intubators use the standard blade, just like they learned to use right handed scissors and other tools when they were kids. It's just a matter of practice.

Problems with Techniques

As mentioned earlier, a blade placed in the center of the tongue produces a mound of tissue that blocks the view (Fig. 5-4). Make sure that

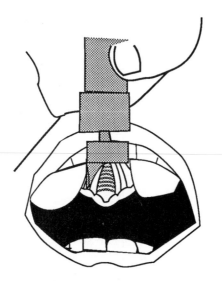

Fig. 5-4. The tongue will get in the way if you place the blade in the middle.

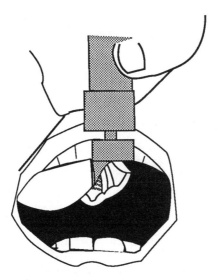

Fig. 5-5. Push the blade as far to the left as possible or there won't be room to pass the tube.

you slide the blade as far to the left side of the mouth as you can. This gets the tongue out of your way. It also places the blade close to the midline, a very stable position for lifting and balancing the head.

Leaving the blade too far to the right often gives you an excellent view of the cords but no room to pass the tube (Fig. 5-5). Sometimes you can't even get the tube into the mouth. This may be your problem if you routinely ask an assistant to pull the right corner of the mouth out of the way.

Sometimes you have a great view with a straight blade but can't pass the tube. Straight Miller blades have the light bulb on the right. When this light bulb is angled toward the right it often deflects the endotracheal tube. If you simply rotate the blade slightly to the left, you will raise the bulb out of the way (Fig. 5-6).

The other common error with a straight blade is inserting it too deep, into the esophagus. If you can't identify any landmarks, slowly pull the blade back. Often the larynx will fall into view. A straight

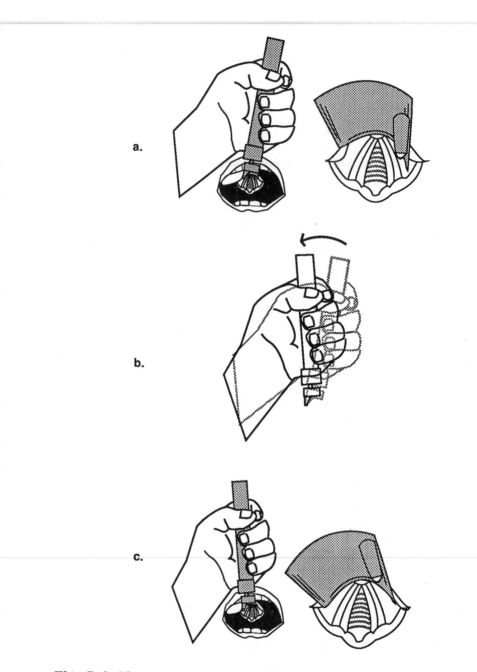

Fig. 5-6. If you can see the cords, but the light bulb deflects your tube, as in **a**, then rotate your hand slightly to the left as in **b**. This often allows the tube to pass without difficulty.

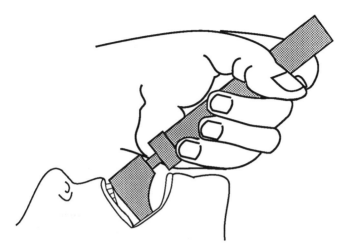

Fig. 5-7. Don't push on the teeth. Lift upward instead. Like tennis: keep the wrist stiff and the elbow straight.

blade can "tent" the esophagus and make it look like vocal cords if you haven't actually seen both.

Failure to lift the lower jaw upward is another common error. Inexperienced intubators place their blade very gently, and then barely lift the jaw. They fear hurting the patient. They don't realize that unless they lift the epiglottis and tongue up, they will see nothing. This leads to the next error. Failing to see anything, they then use the blade like a lever to lift the epiglottis. The only fulcrum available is the front row of teeth (Fig. 5-7). This is very dangerous for the teeth. Never lever on the teeth. Always lift. Properly done, you will actually lift the head off the bed. This won't hurt the patient.

Edentulous or partially edentulous people frequently fool the intubator into thinking he or she has lifted enough. Without teeth you see a great view of the larynx without lifting the jaw. Without the lift, however, the mouth is barely wide enough to pass the tube (Fig. 5-8). Always remember to lift.

Once you have an understanding of the intubation procedure and the purpose of each step, you can easily avoid the common errors.

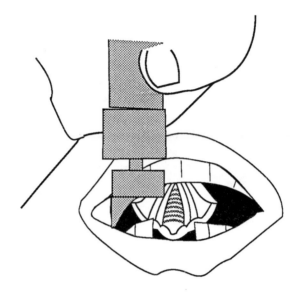

Fig. 5-8. You can see the larynx because the teeth are missing, even though the mouth is not wide enough to pass the tube.

6

Tests for Tube Placement

A fter intubation, check immediately that the tube is positioned correctly in the trachea and not in the esophagus or mainstem bronchus (Fig. 6-1, 6-2). Even expert intubators occasionally intubate the esophagus. This is not a problem as long as you recognize the error and correct it at once.

Seven Steps for Correct Tube Placement

One of the first ways to be sure of tube placement is to see the endotracheal tube between the vocal cords. As you start to remove your laryngoscope blade look for the cords. Remove the blade slowly. Carefully hold the endotracheal tube to avoid pulling the tube out with the blade. Now perform the following tests.

1. Listen over both sides of the chest for the presence of

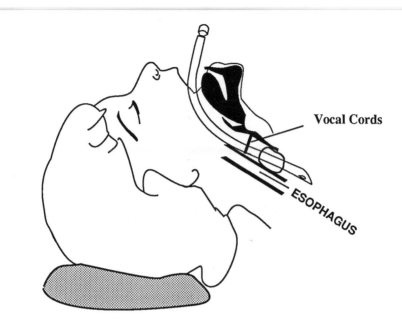

Vocal Cords

ESOPHAGUS

Fig. 6-2. Correct position of the endotracheal tube.

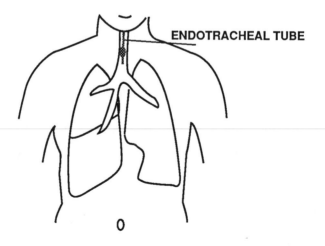

ENDOTRACHEAL TUBE

O

Fig. 6-2. Proper positioning of endotracheal tube above carina.

breath sounds. A tube placed too far down the trachea will lie in one mainstem bronchus and block the other. In this case you will hear breath sounds only on one side of the chest.

2. Listen over the stomach with a stethoscope for a gurgling sound when you ventilate with your bag. This indicates an esophageal intubation.

3. Look for condensation forming inside the tube with each breath. This indicates tracheal placement.

4. Watch for the chest to rise each time you give a breath.

5. If the patient is awake and the cuff is up, he or she will no longer be able to speak.

6. If breathing spontaneously, you will feel air movement with your hand placed over the tube.

7. If you have an end-tidal CO_2 apparatus, attach it and turn it on. CO_2 won't be present with an esophageal intubation.

Esophageal Intubations

Gurgling over the stomach and lack of breath sounds over the chest means the tube is in the esophagus. Calmly remove the tube, having your suction ready. Removal of a tube from the esophagus can cause either passive regurgitation or active vomiting so prepare for this. Next, ventilate the patient by mask until you are feel that the patient is adequately oxygenated. The color of the lips, nail beds, and conjunctivae of the eyes are pink if the patient is oxygenated. Try again. I tell a helper, if I have one, to provide cricoid pressure after removing the tube. The risk of passive regurgitation is higher due to the increased volume of air now in the stomach. Also the passage of the tube into the esophagus opens the sphincters and may decrease their tone. I maintain cricoid pressure until after I place the final tube in the trachea.

Usually there's no doubt about whether the tube lies in the trachea or the esophagus. Unfortunately, there are rare instances when you can't easily tell. It's important to know that you can occasionally hear breath sounds over the chest with an esophageal intubation. These breath sounds, however, will be extremely faint and muffled. The chest will rise poorly. Lung compliance, or the ease of inflating the lungs, will be extremely poor. Condensation does not form inside the tube with each breath. It will be hard to keep your bag filled with gas.

The absence of gurgles over the stomach is not fail-safe. I have seen one case where the stomach was distended with air. The tube cuff effectively sealed the esophagus and there were no audible gurgles over the stomach. We heard faint breath sounds and we were easily able to keep the bag filled with gas because the esophagus was sealed. We suspected esophageal placement because the compliance was extremely poor. Checking the position of the tube with a laryngoscope notified us of its misplacement before injury to the patient occured.

In comparison, patients with severe bronchospasm start with extremely faint breath sounds and very stiff lung compliance. Their chest barely rises. The endotracheal tube may be correctly placed but you sometimes can't tell by listening to the chest alone. Children, on the other hand, have breath sounds that on occasion seem audible over the big toe. You might hear faint "breath" sounds in children with an esophageal intubation.

These real life situations make detection of esophageal intubations more difficult. If you have any doubts about the correct placement of your endotracheal tube *don't hesitate to look with your laryngoscope.*

Having and using an end-tidal CO_2 measuring apparatus will detect all esophageal intubations. The presence of CO_2 in the exhalate can only mean placement of the tube in the trachea. If you are fortunate enough to have such a machine available, you should learn to use it.

Mainstem Intubation

A mainstem intubation occurs when the endotracheal tube extends down one mainstem bronchus, ventilating one lung but obstructing the other (Fig. 6-3). Usually the tube advances down the right side because the right mainstem bronchus is straighter. Louder breath sounds on one side of the chest may mean a mainstem intubation. To cure a mainstem intubation, pull the tube back until you hear breath sounds on both sides of the chest. Secure the tube to prevent it from sliding back down the trachea.

One word of caution. Before you reposition the tube look at the numbers and see if the depth of insertion is correct for that particular patient. This depth is about 21 cm at the teeth in a woman, 22 cm in a man. For a child, determine the depth in cm by dividing the age in years by 2 and then adding 12. If the depth seems correct ask yourself whether another reason for unequal breath sounds exists. Pneumothorax, pneumonectomy, or pleural effusion also cause unequal breath sounds. If the answer is no, then slowly back the tube out until you hear equal breath sounds. However, if the breath sounds do not become equal as the tube gets shallower, stop. Recheck the depth of tube placement by laryngoscopy (to ensure the cuff is below the cords), get an X-ray, and look for other reasons for inequality.

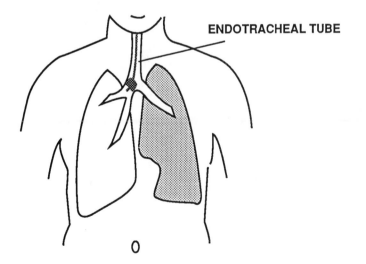

ENDOTRACHEAL TUBE

0

Fig. 6-3. Right Mainstem Intubation Shaded Lung Not Ventilated.

Tube Is Too Shallow

Sometimes after inflating your tube cuff you'll notice a persistent leak. Adding more air to the cuff might make the leak worse. There are two possibilities. The first is that the cuff has a hole in it or that the pilot balloon leaks. In both of these situations the pilot balloon is soft when you squeeze it. The second possibility is that the cuff is above the vocal cords (Fig. 6-4). You can ventilate the patient because the tube tip lies in the trachea, but the cuff can't totally seal the leak. Suspect a cuff above the cords if you can't get rid of a leak, the pilot balloon is tense, and the tube is shallow. Repeat laryngoscopy can differentiate the two.

Further Reading

Pollard BJ, James B: Accidental intubation of the esophagus. *Anaes. Intens. Care* 1980; 8: 183

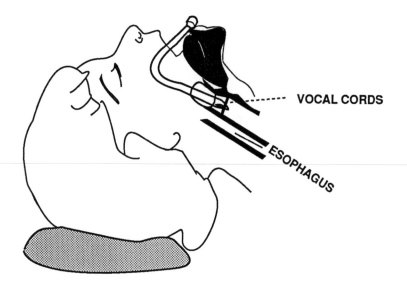

VOCAL CORDS

ESOPHAGUS

Fig. 6-4. Tube bowed in the posterior pharynx, cuff is above the cords.

7

Intubating the Child

Pediatric Airways Differ from Adult Airways

The pediatric airway differs in many ways from that of the adult airway, differences you must recognize to successfully intubate children. Compare the anatomy of a child in Figures 7-1 and 7-2 with the anatomy of an adult in Figures 1-1 and 1-2 (pp. 4 and 5). Table 7-1 summarizes these differences.

Again we have to go back to mechanical advantage to understand why these differences force us to alter our intubation technique. Note that infants differ the most from the adult and that these differences slowly diminish as the child ages. In other words, the older the child, the more like an adult he or she becomes for intubation.

First, to be simplistic, everything in the pediatric airway is smaller, making manipulations with adult hands and equipment technically more difficult.

Second, the cartilage is very soft and pliable. Cricoid pressure or

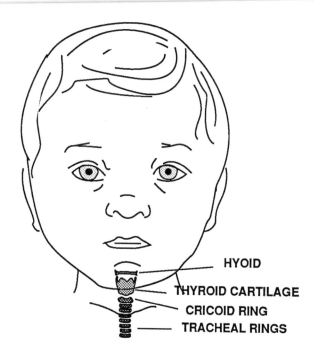

HYOID

THYROID CARTILAGE

CRICOID RING

TRACHEAL RINGS

Fig. 7-1. Notice how much higher in the neck the larynx lies in the infant.

extremes of head position can cause actual obstruction of the airway. For example, over extension of the head may pinch the airway and make passage of the endotracheal tube impossible. It's important to know that over extension or flexion of the head can make spontaneous or assisted ventilation difficult. Reassess the degree of head flexion or extension if you have trouble ventilating the child.

Children have pronounced occiputs, almost a built-in sniffing position. I rarely use a towel under the head of a child less than 9 years old for intubation. Small infants sometimes have too much "sniffing position." Their heads flex on their necks when laying flat on the table. Placing a small towel under such an infant's back corrects the angle of approach.

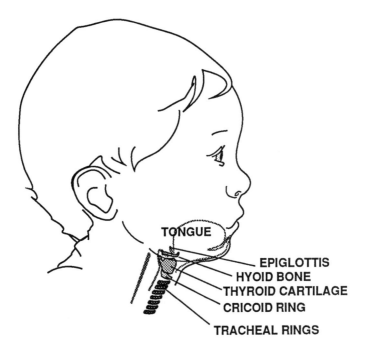

TONGUE
EPIGLOTTIS
HYOID BONE
THYROID CARTILAGE
CRICOID RING
TRACHEAL RINGS

Fig. 7-2. The tongue is large relative to the jaw. The neck is short. The larynx is easily obstructed.

A tongue that is larger relative to the size of the mouth gives us less room to work. It is more difficult to sweep the tongue to the left and displace it forward. The smaller separation between the hyoid and the thyroid cartilage also makes displacing the tongue and associated structures forward more difficult. For these reasons we most frequently choose a straight blade for intubating children.

Using a curved blade in the vallecula often folds the epiglottis down over the vocal cords, blocking the view (Fig. 7-3). The higher anatomical position of the larynx in the neck causes this. However, the angles are such that picking up the epiglottis with the straight blade creates a clear passage.

Picking up the epiglottis in a child of less than five years old can be difficult due to its short, stiff, "U" shaped form. Meticulous placement of the tip of the blade is necessary.

Table 7-1. Comparing Infant and Adult Airways.

	Infant	Adult
Tongue	relatively larger	relatively smaller
Larynx	opposite 2nd and 3rd cervical vertebrae	opposite 4th, 5th, and 6th cervical vertebrae
Epiglottis	"U" shaped, short, stiff	flat, flexible, erect
Hyoid/Thyroid separation	very close	further apart
Glottis	1/2 cartilage	1/4 cartilage
Arytenoids	inclined inferiorly	horizontal
Vocal Cords	concave	horizontal
Cricoid	plate forms funnel	plate vertical
Smallest Diameter	cricoid ring	vocal cord aperture
Consistency of Cartilage	soft	firm
Shape of Head	pronounced occiput	flatter occiput

The arytenoids in the child incline inferiorly, which means the cords slant with their anterior attachment lower than their posterior one. The cords in the adult are horizontal. Because of this slant, the pediatric tube can hang up on the anterior commissure when passing it into the larynx. You can see the tube entering the larynx, it simply refuses to pass. Rotating the tube to the right or left allows the tube to slip off the anterior commissure and pass. Be careful, however, that your tube is

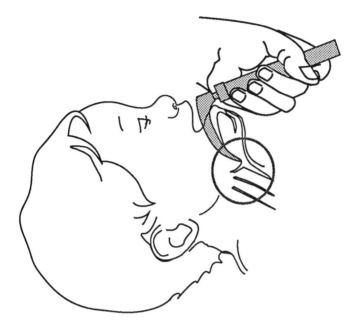

Fig. 7-3. A curved blade will sometimes fold the epiglottis down, hiding your view of the vocal cords.

not too large . If rotation of the tube does not work, remove the tube and try a smaller size. Never force it through.

The vocal cords in the child have a concave upward shape, rather than the horizontal shape of the adult. While this doesn't affect our ability to intubate the child, it can affect our ability to ventilate him. We often use positive pressure with bag and mask to treat a partial airway obstruction or laryngospasm. This works because the positive pressure pushes the vocal cords down, and slightly apart. Once the cords separate even a little bit, the positive pressure expands the space below them. This forces the arytenoids apart, opening the airway. Thinking mechanically, horizontal cords should separate more easily under positive pressure than concave cords, which might overlap more forcefully. To break laryngospasm in the child, we combine positive pressure with chin thrust. Thrusting the chin forward puts tension on the arytenoids and pulls them apart. The gap produced allows pressurization of the space below and the spasm usually breaks.

The cricoid ring is the smallest diameter of the child's airway. In adults the smallest diameter lies between the vocal cords. This means that a tube too large for the child might pass through the vocal cords but not the cricoid ring. Never force an endotracheal tube down a pediatric airway. If the tube will not pass easily, choose a smaller size.

Be gentle in all of your manipulations. Pediatric airways are small and delicate and as such are prone to edema. A comparison to the adult illustrates the relative danger. The typical adult airway is 8 mm in diameter or greater. One mm of circumferential edema from intubation trauma leaves an airway of 6 mm diameter, a 25% reduction. An infant's airway typically is 3 mm in diameter. One mm circumferential edema here leaves an airway 1 mm in diameter, a 68% reduction. Even minimal trauma can create life threatening airway obstruction.

Equipment for Pediatric Intubation

You will need the same type of equipment for the pediatric as for the adult intubation. The main difference to recognize is that the younger children are, the more different their anatomy is from the adult.

Pediatric carts need Miller blades in sizes 0 (premature), 1 (infant), and 2 (child). You can intubate a small child using a large blade, even an adult blade, by inserting the blade to the minimum depth needed to see the larynx. When using such a large blade you must shift the tongue to the left as far as possible. Otherwise the blade will fill the small mouth and leave you with no room to maneuver. Intubating a larger child with a blade that is too short may be impossible. Always try to have the correct size blade available for use.

Oral and nasal airways also come in assorted sizes. While not needed for the intubation itself, you should always have the correct size available for the child. Unexpected difficulties in intubation may arise. You need a large suction catheter for clearing the mouth of secretions and vomit. You also need one which will go down the smallest endotracheal tube you might use.

Predict the correct size endotracheal tube before you start the intubation. Have both the next larger and next smaller sizes available in case you need them (Table 7-2).

Table 7-2. Suggested sizes for pediatric endotracheal tubes:

Age	Size
Premature	2.5-3.5 mm I.D.
Newborn	3.5 mm I.D.
3-12 months	4.0 mm I.D.
1-2 years	4.5 mm I.D.
over 2 years	4.5 + (age in years ÷ 4)
French size, over 2 years	age in years + 18
Insertion depth to mid trachea	12 + (age in years ÷ 2)

We don't routinely use cuffed endotracheal tubes in children less than about 9 years old. Children's airways are small and cuffs take up space. Avoiding cuffs allows the use of a larger diameter tube, thereby minimizing airway resistance and maximizing airway toilet. It also avoids the excess pressure on the mucosa that a cuff can cause.

Do you need to worry about aspiration? In the young child, the smallest diameter is the cricoid ring, a round hole. Therefore the proper size round tube should seal the larynx and prevent aspiration. In the adult, the smallest diameter is the triangular opening between the cords. Our adult tube needs a cuff to help seal off the surrounding space. A properly sized pediatric tube will allow an air leak at 15-20 cm of water pressure but will sustain a seal below this. The absence of a leak means too large a tube, which may cause mucosal trauma and edema. The presence of a leak below 15-20 cm water pressure means too small a tube, increasing the risk of aspiration and possibly inadequate ventilation.

Intubating the Infant

The infant's head lies naturally in the sniffing position due to the prominence of the occiput. In fact, sometimes the occiput seems too high. The larynx falls too low to see easily. In such cases place a small hand towel or similar thickness object underneath the infant's shoulders. This raises the rest of the body and straightens the airway. The occiput tends to roll in the infant, making the act of balancing the head on your blade a challenge. Don't hesitate to have an assistant hold the head for you if you have problems. A small "donut" under the head or rolled towel placed on either side of the head serves the same purpose. With practice, balancing the head becomes second nature.

Open the mouth with your right index finger and thumb as far to the right side of the mouth as possible. Extend the head slightly as you do so. Avoid hyperextension which can obstruct the infant airway. The infant's mouth is so small compared to your hand that failure to place your fingers on the right will block your view. It can prevent insertion of the blade.

Carefully insert your blade into the child's mouth with your left hand and advance the blade until you see the epiglottis. Pick up the epiglottis gently with your blade and lift the mandible upward (Fig. 7-4). Sweep the tongue to the left as you do so. Avoid pressing on the upper gum line as you lift. The infant tongue is much larger relative to the mouth and mandible than the adult. Failure to sweep the tongue to the left will leave no room for visualization or for passage of the tube. A common error in children is to insert the blade too deep, into the esophagus. If you cannot see anatomy that you recognize then gently

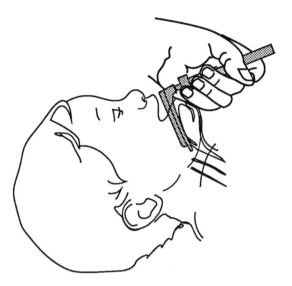

Fig. 7-4. Place head in neutral position.

and under direct vision pull the blade tip back. Often the larynx will fall into view.

Figure 7-5 demonstrates a way for you to provide your own cricoid pressure and manipulation of the trachea of a small infant. Use your fifth or little finger to gently push the larynx into position as you lift.

Pick up the chosen tube with the right hand and pass it through the vocal cords as you are watching. *Stop when you see the double ring marking pass the cords.* Carefully remove your laryngoscope blade. Be sure that the tube lies in the trachea by listening to the chest as described earlier. The small size of the infant allows easy transmission of sound. As my teachers used to say, you can hear breath sounds over a child's foot. Therefore, be especially careful to listen over the stomach and the chest to be certain that the tube is down the right hole.

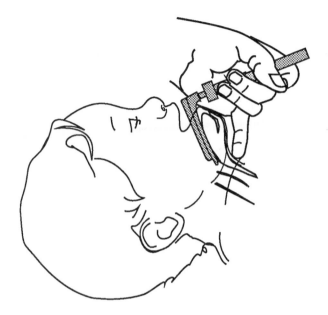

Fig. 7-5. Applying cricoid pressure using the little finger.

Another important factor is that the trachea of the infant is very short. Mainstem intubation is easy and fairly common. Make sure that you hear breath sounds on both sides of the chest before and after you secure the tube. Can you see the chest move on both sides? Note the depth marking on the tube in relationship to the gum line and compare it to the calculated depth. The infant trachea is so short compared to the adult that changing the head position can lead to a mainstem intubation or an extubation. Raising the chin raises the tube away from the carina, lowering the chin lowers the tube toward the carina. "The hose follows the nose" is a useful mnemonic.

Infants can't hold their breaths as long as an adult can before the onset of hypoxia. Their functional residual capacity, that part of the lung storing oxygen, is small relative to their body size. Their metabolic rate is almost double that of an adult. If you experience difficulty with the intubation of an infant, stop the intubation and ventilate the child before proceeding with another attempt. *Lack of ventilation hurts patients, not the lack of an endotracheal tube.*

Intubating the Child

Gather the appropriate sizes of laryngoscope blades, endotracheal tubes, and ancillary equipment before approaching the child. Having it available before you start allows for greater flexibility and faster intubation.

Most children younger than 9 years old do not need a head roll to lift them into the sniffing position. However, look at the child and individualize the need based on the child's anatomy. You now know the angles that you need to bring the airway into a straight line.

The older the child, the more like an adult he or she will be. The child has some additional problems, however, that the infant lacks.

Children frequently have enlarged tonsils and adenoids. The tonsils sometimes meet or "kiss" in the midline and make visualization of the larynx a challenge. When faced with "kissing" tonsils, take your time while placing the laryngoscope blade. Avoid traumatizing the posterior pharynx. Tonsils are very friable tissue and can bleed easily.

If you can't intubate with the first attempt, withdraw, ventilate the child, and try again. You may need an oral airway to adequately ventilate these children. The tonsillar and adenoidal tissue fills the "dead space" in the nose and posterior pharynx and can cause partial obstruction. Nasal airways can cause nosebleeds in children with hypertrophied adenoids. I only use them in these children as a last resort. Lubricate the nasal airway well before insertion and be gentle as you pass it. Adenoidal tissue can plug nasal airways, as well as nasal endotracheal tubes, after passing through the nose. This creates the risk of obstruction or of aspiration of tissue. Pass a suction catheter through the tube while the tip still lies in the posterior pharynx to clear it before pushing it further into the trachea.

Another way to establish an airway is to hold the mouth open under the mask. I use the hand grip shown in Fig. 7-6a, b. This mimics the action of an oral airway.

a.

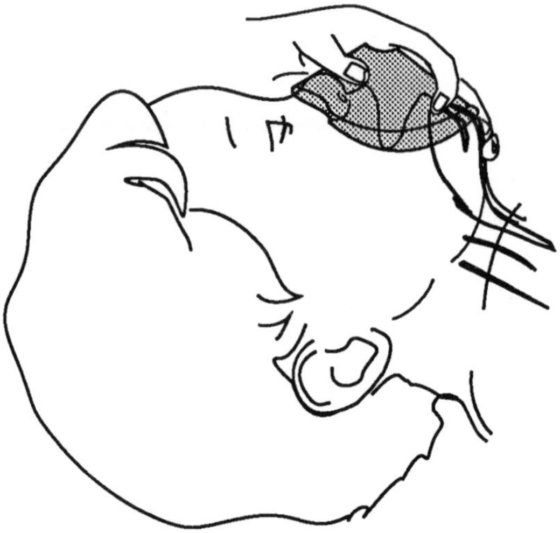

b.

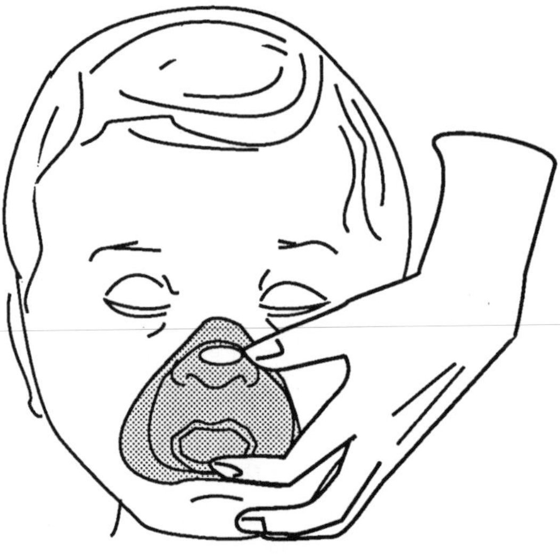

Fig. 7-6a,b. Technique to hold the mouth open under the mask. Pull lower jaw upward and toward the feet by hooking the lower fingers under the mandible. Maintain the seal with your thumb and index finger.

Children differ from infants in having teeth, often in various stages of attachment. If you have the time, always look for loose or missing teeth before you start. Forewarned is forearmed. Check for missing teeth after you finish. You should look for any teeth that are newly missing. Often the tooth will lie in the posterior pharynx. If it isn't there, you should take an X-ray to be sure that the tooth isn't in the trachea or obstructing a bronchus. A tooth in the stomach will eventually pass.

The basic thing to remember when intubating a child is that the child is not a miniature adult. The anatomy and the physiologic responses to stress are different. Always take these factors into account when you approach a child. You'll make intubation easier and safer for all concerned.

Further Reading

Browning DH, Graves SA: Incidence of aspiration with endotracheal tubes in children. *J. Pediatr.* 1983; 102: 582

Koka BV, Jeon JM, et.al.: Postextubation croup in children. *Anesth. Analg.* 1977; 56: 501

Gregory GA: *Pediatric Anesthesia.* New York. Churchill-Livingstone, 1983, 437-439

8

Studies in Difficult Intubations: Tricks of the Trade

Most intubations proceed without difficulty. Certain patients, however, are difficult to intubate by virtue of their anatomy or the circumstances of the intubation. Unfortunately, such patients can also be difficult to ventilate, creating a double quandary. With experience you learn to anticipate these difficult intubations. This allows you to avoid problems by altering technique at the start. Let's look at some of the more common difficult intubations and some of the tricks of the trade. I'll describe some of the special techniques for manually ventilating these patients as we proceed.

One word of caution. Difficulty in intubation, especially when accompanied by difficulty in ventilation, is a life threatening situation. Even experienced intubators seek help when they have trouble. Inexperienced intubators are well advised to have an experienced intubator standing by during the intubation. This can save precious time in an emergency. The more experienced person can also give you pointers on correcting your technique.

Cardiac Arrest

Cardiac arrest victims are often challenging intubations because of the circumstances surrounding the intubation. Excitement and apprehension accompany this life saving effort. If you don't intubate very often, you'll be very nervous. Even experienced intubators get excited in emergency situations. We control our excitement and let the adrenalin work for us rather than against us. **Step one**, therefore, is to remain in control of your own excitement.

Step two is to quickly assess the situation. Is the patient being ventilated? Is there suction available? What help do you have? What position is the patient in and how can you optimize that position?

You usually find the patient in one of two awkward positions. When the patient lies on the floor, you must intubate on your knees. Mechanical advantage is more difficult from this position. You must rely more heavily on your arm strength to lift the head rather than your upper back and shoulder muscles. The natural tendency to lean forward and bend your arm will make it hard for you to balance (Fig. 8-1).

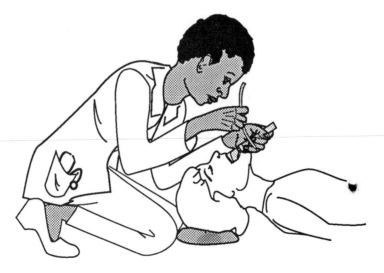

Fig. 8-1. Awkward positioning of intubator makes for difficult intubations.

The weight of the patient pulls you forward when you try to lift. Instead, keep your left arm and your back as straight as you can. Tense your buttocks and thigh muscles to form a firm base of support, and lift upward (Fig. 8-2). Remember that several folded sheets or towels under the head lift it into the sniffing position. Ask for help in lifting the head into position if you need it. Your head and shoulders should be over the patient's head. This improves your center of gravity during the lift.

Some anesthesiologists recommend lying prone on your stomach to intubate a patient on the floor. They place their weight on their elbows, eliminating the problem of balance and improving the angle of view.

Unfortunately, the second awkward position finds the patient in the typical hospital bed (Fig. 8-3, 8-4). Why is this awkward? First,

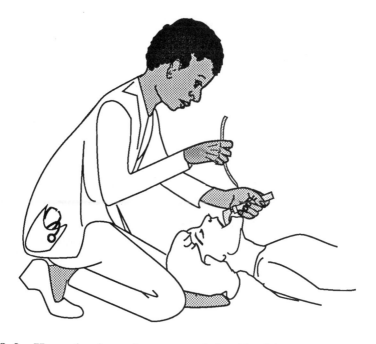

Fig. 8-2. Keep back and arm straight. Position your center of gravity over the patient's head.

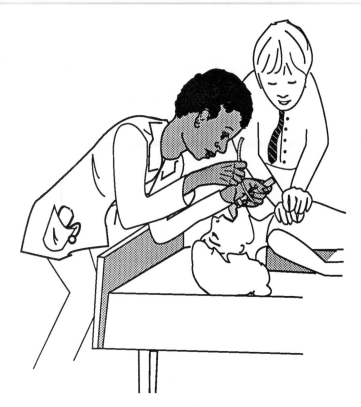

Fig. 8-3. The problems with intubation in the bed: awkward angle, headboard in the way, backboard makes head angle severe, CPR moves the patient.

most hospital beds have a fairly high headboard which prevents easy access to the patient's head. Have someone remove this headboard while you prepare your equipment.

Second, if you can't easily reach the patient, pull him or her toward the head of the bed. This only takes a moment, but for small individuals like myself it is a moment well spent. If you do not have to lean forward you will have more effective mechanical advantage and control.

Third, you will often find the patient on a soft hospital mattress with the hard cardiac arrest board under his back. Because this allows

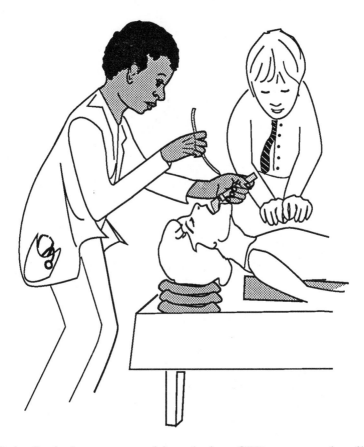

Fig. 8-4. Optimize your position during CPR: remove headboard, move patient closer to head of bed, place head in sniffing position, stop CPR during attempt, keep back and arm straight.

effective CPR, we take this position for granted. We often fail to notice that the patient's head now hangs fully extended off the back of the board. A look at the angles that this produces shows that you must lift the patient's head much higher to straighten the airway (Fig. 8-5). Lifting a heavy head high under these conditions is quite difficult. Use pillows to put the head in the sniffing position and decrease the lift you need. Don't hesitate to ask for assistance in lifting or in maintaining lift

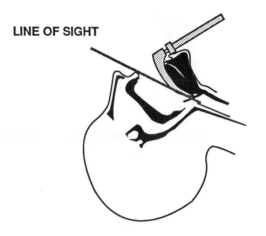

LINE OF SIGHT

Fig. 8-5. Overextension of the head makes the larynx appear more anterior on laryngoscopy.

while you place the tube. Cricoid pressure to push the larynx down into view can also help in situations like this (Fig. 8-6, 8-7).

Fourth, CPR means that someone is forcefully pushing on the patient's chest. The patient and bed are both moving up and down. Moving targets are hard to hit at the best of times. I usually get in position, visualize the larynx, and try to pass the tube. If the movement prevents this, I ask for momentary discontinuation of CPR. Yell "stop CPR." Pass the tube. Yell "begin CPR." This should take no longer than 15 to 20 seconds, usually less. If you have any difficulty passing the tube have your associates begin CPR again. Remove your blade, and ventilate the patient. Try again. Never delay CPR for an extended period because of an intubation attempt.

Always remember that adequate ventilation is more important than intubation. If you have difficulty, stop and ventilate the patient while you decide what you must try next.

Following intubation, suction the tube and trachea carefully to remove any secretions and blood aspirated during the resuscitation.

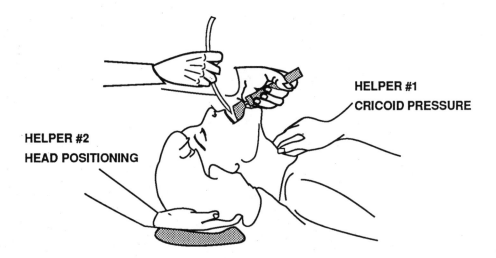

HELPER #1
CRICOID PRESSURE

HELPER #2
HEAD POSITIONING

Fig. 8-6. The use of helpers.

Obesity

Patients with obesity or with short, muscular necks can sometimes be hard to intubate (Fig. 8-8). Excess soft tissue around the larynx and decreased hyoid/mentum distance hinder displacement of those tissues forward by the laryngoscope blade. Without such displacement the larynx may not be visible. Excess soft tissue collapsing over the laryngeal structures may make manual ventilation difficult.

Try placing an oral or nasal airway if you have trouble ventilating this type of patient. Frequently this is all you need to do. Ask for an assistant if obstruction persists. Use both of your hands to obtain a good seal on the mask (Fig. 8-9). Place one hand on either side of the head. Place thumbs on the top of the mask, index fingers on the bottom and hook your middle fingers underneath the angle of the mandible. Pull up forcefully. With this movement you shift the mandible forward and pull the obstructing tissue up and off the larynx. Your assistant can now squeeze the ventilation bag. When using this technique, be sure that your assistant is adequately ventilating the patient.

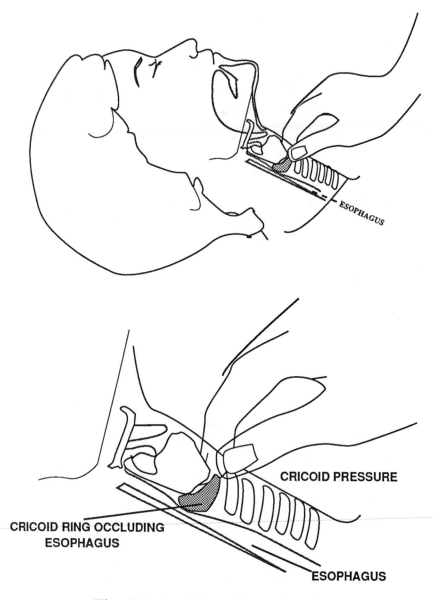

Fig. 8-7. Applying cricoid pressure.

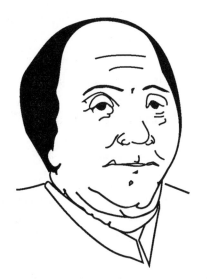

Fig. 8-8. The obese patient often has a short, thick neck and much tissue under the skin.

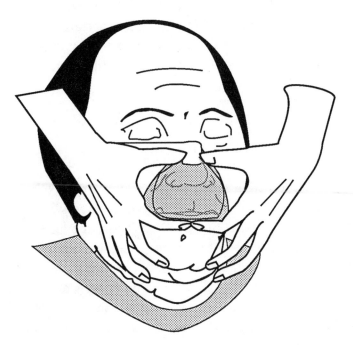

Fig. 8-9. Using both of your hands to get a good mask seal.

Watch the chest rise, see the air condense on the mask if it is clear, and have someone listen for breath sounds.

With ventilation now assured, you can worry about the intubation. I usually make the first attempt at intubation with the blade I am most comfortable with. In emergency situations I often choose a Macintosh curved blade. In my opinion, its broader flange is more forgiving of less than perfect placement and awkward positioning — conditions common in the emergency. It also makes balancing the patient's head easier in those circumstances. However, in obese patients or those with an " anterior" airway, the curved blade sometimes won't give you good visualization. It doesn't allow enough displacement of tissue forward in these cases and the larynx remains hidden. Therefore, if I can't see the larynx with the Mac on the first try in this patient group, then I switch to a straight blade. The straight blade doesn't rely as heavily on the ability to displace the tissues of the hypopharynx forward. It flattens them.

The straight blade has another advantage. Inserting the curved blade can be difficult in the obese patient because the chest can get in the way of the handle. The straight blade bypasses this problem. Substituting a short laryngoscope handle often works as well.

Through the Veil:
Partial Plates and Cleft Palates

Patients will sometimes have missing upper front teeth. These patients pose a peculiar problem for intubation. Beginners frequently get a superb view of the larynx, they just can't pass the tube. The absence of teeth allows the intubator to see the larynx without lifting the mandible (Fig. 8-10). Because they have not opened the patient's mouth enough they can't get the tube past the teeth on either side. The solution is to lift the jaw upward even after you can see the larynx. Don't try to pass the tube through the gap. There usually is not enough space.

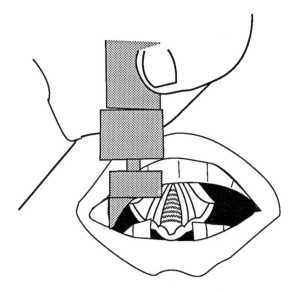

Fig. 8-10. You can see the larynx because the teeth are missing, even though the mouth is not wide enough to pass the tube.

Edentulous

The same situation described above can occur here. You see the larynx before the mouth is open wide enough to allow passage of the tube. The absence of teeth on the mandible sometimes changes the angle of the blade during lift. Usually, however, the change in "feel" and balance that this produces is minimal. It is often offset by the relief of the intubator about not having to worry about the teeth. Intubation is easier without teeth if you lift enough.

However, ventilation of the edentulous patient often causes problems. Sealing the mask without the teeth to give support to the cheeks and form to the mouth is challenging. I find the newer, low dead space masks with an inflated cuff around the edge easiest to use. They conform to the loose contour of the face with less tendency to allow gaps and air leaks. However, even these masks occasionally fail.

When gaps occur they are usually over the bridge of the nose or on the side opposite the hand holding the mask. With the left hand holding the mask, the leak usually appears on the right side. First, simply allow the weight of your ventilation bag and attachments to push down the mask help obtain a seal. Turn the apparatus on the connector until its weight is centered over the leak. If this doesn't work, try plugging the leak with a piece of gauze under the mask. An assistant can help push cheek tissue up over the mask edge at the site of the leak or leaks.

If the above fails, try a variation on the two handed technique I described for the obese patient (Fig. 8-11). Place your thumbs on the top of the mask, your index fingers on the bottom. Use your middle and ring fingers to bunch the cheek tissue up to seal the mask on either side. This leaves your fifth fingers free to hook under the mandible and lift. Your assistant ventilates.

You can use the weight of your own chin over the bridge of the mask to stop leaks here (Fig. 8-12). While the position sounds awkward,

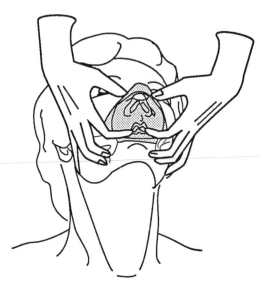

Fig. 8-11. A method to seal mask leaks using your middle and fourth fingers to push the cheek against the mask.

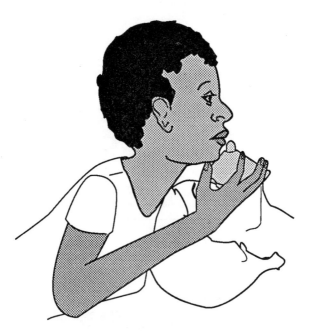

Fig. 8-12. One technique to maintain a good seal with a leak over the nose. In the absence of helpers pressure from your own chin can press the mask down over the nose. One hand helps seal. The other one ventilates the patient as needed.

it does allow you to ventilate the patient fairly well. I often use it in the absence of assistants to help me.

Another trick consists of placing an infant-sized Rendall-Baker mask in the patient's mouth — under the cheeks but outside the gums. This recreates the form and support of the missing teeth. The mask fits over the mouth and cheeks without leaks. The hole in the pediatric mask lets you ventilate (Fig. 8-13).

Receding Chins

Patients with receding chins, caused by hypoplastic mandibles, often have very "anterior airways" (Fig. 8-14). There is frequently not

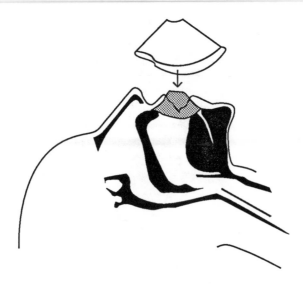

Fig. 8-13. In edentulous patients you can place an infant mask inside the cheeks on top of the gums. An adult mask fits over the cheeks and usually seals well.

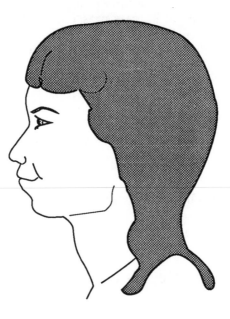

Fig. 8-14. Patients with hypoplastic mandibles, or receding chins, often have very anterior larynxes.

enough room to displace the tissue forward when you intubate. You may need to do an awake intubation if the chin is extremely hypoplastic. You should anticipate the need for cricoid pressure and a straight blade.

Overbites

The upper teeth in a prominent overbite will get in the way of a Macintosh blade (Fig. 8-15). You must follow the curve of the tongue into the mouth to insert a curved blade. The higher vertical profile of this blade may bump into the teeth if you don't open the mouth as much as possible. Straight blades avoid these problems.

Lift straight upward on these patients. You can easily push on the teeth if you use your laryngoscope as a lever. There are two tricks to try if you can't see. The first is cricoid pressure, a handy standby anytime you have difficulty seeing the larynx. The second is to substitute a shorter straight blade. You can sometimes insert a number one two Miller blade inside the mouth such that the radius of any rotational movement of your blade occurs inside the radius of the teeth. This allows

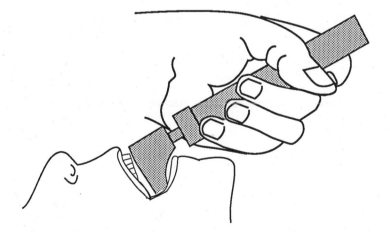

Fig. 8-15. In the presence of an overbite be careful to lift the jaw upward instead of rotating the blade on the teeth.

you to "lever" safely. If the blade is long enough, it can give you a better view.

Poor Neck Mobility

Poor neck mobility can occur for a number of reasons. Arthritic fusion of the vertebrae in older individuals often limits the range of motion. This limitation can be so severe that no extension or flexion of the head can occur. Torticollis or wry neck prevents full range of motion. Finally, trauma to the neck may limit motion. In the latter case your patient may have a cervical collar or other restraint to prevent damage to the spinal cord.

It is often safest to intubate these patient awake. Techniques include the use of fiberoptic laryngoscopes and awake blind-nasal intubations. Sometimes the only safe choice is a tracheostomy. We'll discuss awake intubations later. For the moment let's assume that you have a patient with no neck mobility in need of intubation. He is unconscious or perhaps in cardiac arrest. What can you try?

First, let's discuss the patient with limited range of motion but *no* risk of spinal cord injury. When you can't extend the head you can't align the airway axes. The larynx looks very anterior during laryngoscopy (Fig. 8-16). Sometimes you can't even see the arytenoids. Lift the head as far off the bed as you can, suspending the head from your blade. This may be enough to bring the arytenoids into view. If it is, aim for the space immediately above the arytenoids, where the gap between the vocal cords lies. Straight blades often work better than curved blades in this situation. Forceful cricoid pressure may push the larynx down into view.

Make sure the stylet in your endotracheal tube has a hook on the end, shaping the tube like a hockey stick. Test to make sure that the stylet slides in and out easily despite the hook. Aim your tube anteriorly at the point where you think the larynx lies. Be gentle.

When you put a pronounced bend in the stylet, you sometimes find that the tube will not advance easily. The tip of the tube points upward,

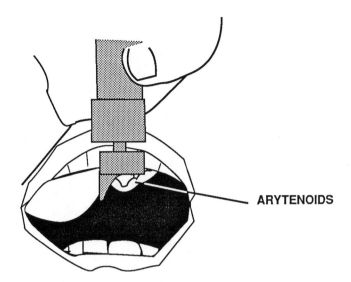

ARYTENOIDS

Fig. 8-16. The view seen with an anterior larynx. Here you can
see the arytenoids. Often you see no landmarks.

into the anterior wall of the trachea (Fig. 8-17). In this case you will
feel resistance to pushing the tube in. Often the assistant holding cricoid pressure feels you pushing against the larynx. If this happens, fix
your tube firmly in position and have someone else slowly remove the
stylet from the tube. Advance the tube gently at the same time. Gently
twisting the tube may allow the bevel to slip off the anterior commissure and slide down the trachea (Fig. 8-18).

If this fails and you feel you have the tube lined up with the laryngeal inlet there is another trick to try. Remove the stylet carefully.
Advance a long and fairly firm suction catheter or nasogastric tube
down the endotracheal tube while you hold it steady. Once inserted,
use the catheter as a stylet to advance the endotracheal tube.

By aiming your tube at the likely location you can sometimes pass
the tube into the larynx without seeing landmarks. If you do pass the
tube blindly, make absolutely certain that you immediately test for
proper tube placement. Tubes can easily slip into the esophagus in situations like this.

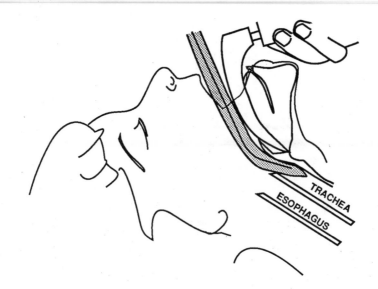

Fig. 8-17. You may not be able to advance the tube if the stylet is bent too sharply. If this happens, slowly back the stylet out — then push the tube forward.

In the event that you can't intubate the patient, ventilate the patient by mask between attempts. Periodically suction the mouth and oropharynx for secretions. Ask for other intubators to try.

What do you do if you absolutely should not or can't flex or extend the patient's neck? When faced with the trauma patient in a halo, cervical collar, or other restraining device you face a difficult responsibility. You must secure the airway without injuring the patient. A halo device will keep the patient's head in a safe position. You may therefore try the techniques described above without further securing the head. Patients secured by sandbags or cervical collars must receive further protection. Have a knowledgeable assistant, preferably the surgeon or neurosurgeon, hold the head and neck in a neutral position while you attempt intubation (Fig 8-19). Lift the mandible upward, *not* the head and neck. Often you can see enough anatomy to allow intubation.

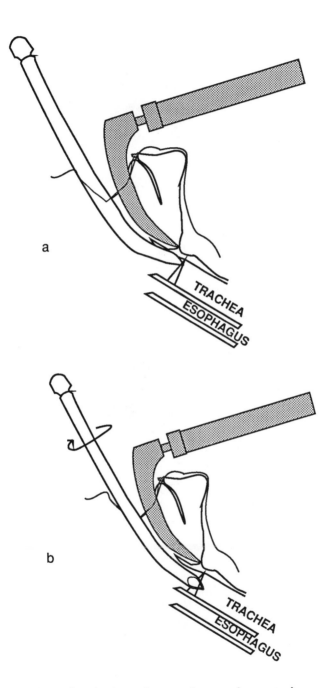

Fig. 8-18. The tube tip in **a** is caught on the anterior commisure. Rotate the tube, as in **b**, to allow it to pass.

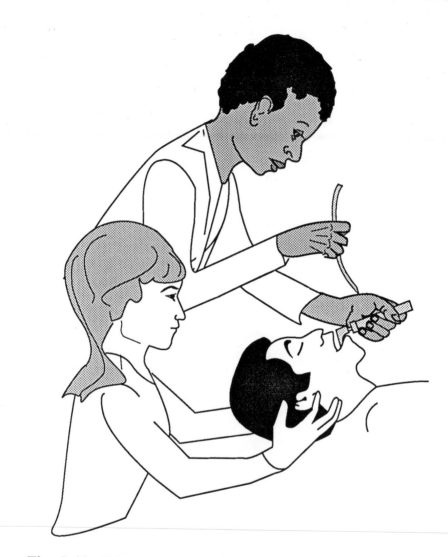

Fig. 8-19. When intubating the patient with possible neck injury have an assistant stabilize the head and neck. Lift only the mandible. Don't extend the head.

If you can't intubate quickly, a tracheostomy may be the quickest and safest means of securing the airway.

Fixed Airway Obstruction

Airway obstruction is a life threatening emergency. Poor intubation technique may worsen airway obstruction, a potentially fatal situation. If you are an inexperienced intubator, you should summon and defer to the skill and judgement of any available experienced intubators. We often bring such patients to an operating room. There they are either intubated awake or under deep inhalational anesthesia with spontaneous ventilation. The personnel and means to perform emergency tracheostomy are immediately available and ready. Inexperienced intubators should not attempt intubation of an obstructed airway unless in their judgement only immediate intubation will save the patient's life.

The most common emergencies involving airway obstruction include epiglottitis, croup, trauma, and tumor. When you initially evaluate these patients let them sit up if they're more comfortable breathing in this position. Give them supplemental oxygen. Someone who can manage airway obstruction must accompany the patient if the patient needs to leave the emergency area. They should *never* be sent for special examinations, X-rays, or another facility, alone. This intubator must take all the equipment needed for intubation and ventilation. Don't subject children to unnecessary laboratory exams or separate them prematurely from parents. Crying and screaming increases airway edema. Keep them calm. *Do not* sedate them. Sedation may cause them to lose what airway they have.

If the patient is dying and can't wait for more specialized help, you must proceed with caution. Call for the means to do cricothyrotomy or tracheostomy. Never paralyze or sedate a patient with airway obstruction. The muscle tone of the larynx may be the only factor maintaining the airway. Gently visualize the larynx by direct laryngoscopy. Patients in extremis usually won't fight you as you do this. If you can identify landmarks, then intubate the patient. Use an endotracheal tube of appropriate size. By appropriate size I mean the largest one that will fit in the swollen airway. Don't try the largest one that should normally fit a patient of that size and age. Have a variety of tubes available, including the smallest pediatric tubes. I once used an infant sized number 3 endotracheal tube to intubate an 80 kg, 72 inch adult with epiglottitis because that was the only tube that would fit.

If you can't identify the anatomy, look for air bubbles coming from the larynx as a clue to the location of the cords. Have an assistant push on the chest if the patient isn't breathing. Give oxygen during the attempts by having an assistant blow oxygen into the mouth. Adequately ventilate with oxygen between attempts.

I advise the lone inexperienced intubator to stop after two or three attempts. Emergency cricothyrotomy or tracheostomy is indicated at this point.

Blood in the Oropharynx

Blood in the oropharynx predisposes the patient to aspiration and hypoxia. Fresh post operative cleft palates and tonsillectomies, trauma victims, and massive G.I. bleeders are examples. In the worst case scenario, the patient is unconscious, unable to protect their airway, and is bleeding so badly that you can't see any landmarks at all. It's a frightening experience.

Handling the situation in an operating room where there is lighting, equipment, personnel, and experienced intubators makes sense. Life threatening emergencies sometimes force less than optimal circumstances.

The patient needs ventilation and oxygen. If they are breathing well on their own give them supplemental oxygen, start intravenous volume replacement, and supply suction for the airway. Ventilate them if they are not breathing adequately. Place these patients in a position that allows the blood to drain away from the airway. For example, place them on their side or sitting up leaning forward. Never let them lay face up and flat. If they must be supine, as during CPR, then place the bed in Trendelenburg to allow the blood to pool in the upper pharynx, away from the airway. Suction the mouth frequently. Turn their face to the side if you can. If you hear gurgling as the patient ventilates, then suction the patient. Patients who can't protect their airways need intubation as quickly as possible.

You can manually ventilate patients on their side. You may need help maintaining the mask seal. Have someone check breath sounds. It is far easier to place the patient left side down. This way the left hand can hold the mask while resting on the bed and the right one can ventilate freely. Right side down points the bag into the bed, forcing you to reverse the equipment (Fig 8-20 a,b).

If the bleeding is serious, you may prefer to intubate the patient on their side (Fig. 8-21). Again, left side down is optimal. Your left hand pushes the tongue to the left during laryngoscopy. With the left side down, gravity helps pull the tongue out of the way. It also leaves plenty of room for your right arm to maneuver the tube. The anatomy is the same and you should not let the different position unnerve you. You won't have the weight of the head pulling it down during laryngoscopy because the head stays on the bed. The blade may pull the head without lifting the jaw. If this is a problem, have a helper hold the head steady as you look.

Inexperienced and experienced intubators alike may prefer a combined method. Place the patient left side down and in slight Trendelenburg to ventilate the patient until everything is ready for intubation. Use cricoid pressure to prevent passive regurgitation of swallowed blood and secretions. Cricoid pressure may not prevent aspiration of the blood pooling in the oropharynx so suction frequently as you wait. Just before intubation clean the airway thoroughly, hand the suction catheter to an assistant, and turn the patient onto their back. Maintain cricoid pressure. Intubate them quickly. Have your assistant suction the airway as you work if needed.

If your first attempt fails use your judgement about turning the patient lateral or keeping him supine. Whichever you choose, suction the

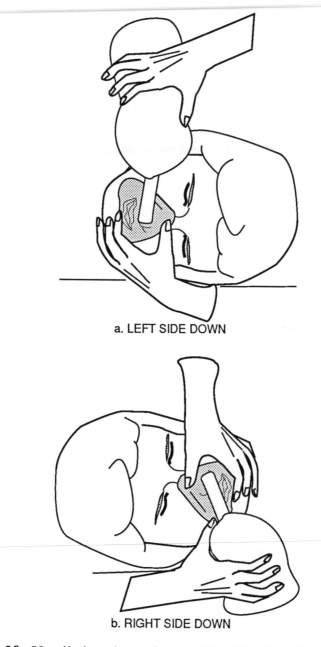

a. LEFT SIDE DOWN

b. RIGHT SIDE DOWN

Fig. 8-20. Ventilating the patient on his side. Ventilation with left side down is easiest. The hand squeezing the bag is free to move. With the right side down, the angle of your hands is awkward and the bag bumps into the bed.

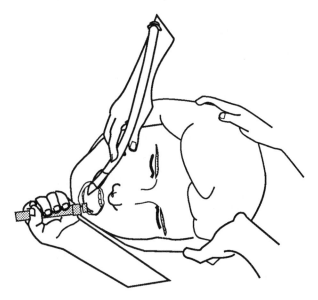

Fig. 8-21. Intubation with the head left side down. Notice helper stabilizing head.

airway well between attempts. When the anatomy is covered in blood, identification of landmarks can be difficult. Look for air bubbles coming from the larynx as a clue to the location of the cords. A gentle, abrupt push on the chest by an assistant can provide bubbles for you if the patient isn't breathing. If the patient is breathing, you will hear breath sounds through the endotracheal tube. These sounds will stop instantly if the tube enters the esophagus. Use the breath sounds as another clue to tube position.

After intubating, thoroughly suction the endotracheal tube as aspiration of blood is very common in these cases. Another danger is that blood left in the tube may clot, obstructing the tube and preventing ventilation.

The Use of Cricoid Pressure

Cricoid pressure is one of the most valuable aides you have during a difficult intubation. We use it not only to improve visualization of the so-called anterior airway, but also to help prevent aspiration. To apply cricoid pressure, place your thumb on one side of the cricoid ring and your index or ring finger on the other. Push down firmly. This forces the cricoid ring against the vertebral column and effectively seals the esophagus. It also forces the vocal cords downward and perhaps into the field of view (see again, Fig. 8-7a, b). You'll frequently use cricoid pressure. However, you should recognize that even this technique has problems.

While very effective against passive regurgitation, you should release cricoid pressure when the patient actively vomits. The obstructed esophagus might rupture because of high pressure.

Also, no matter how useful cricoid pressure usually is, it will occasionally prevent passage of the endotracheal tube. Cricoid pressure will sometimes pinch a child's soft airway closed. Sometimes in an adult the angle created by the downward displacement is too acute, preventing entry of the tube. This is especially true when inexperienced helpers push on other parts of the larynx in addition to the cricoid. If you are having a great deal of difficulty intubating, consider releasing part or all of the cricoid pressure to see if it helps.

A Last Word

The patients described above may prove impossible for even an experienced intubator to intubate. If intubation fails after inducing general anesthesia, we wake the patient up and intubate them awake. If this is not an option and the need for an airway is emergent and life threatening we call for a tracheostomy. As you gain experience as an intubator, you will find many patients who are difficult to intubate. Rarely will you be in a situation where you are the only person trained in intubation.

Never hesitate to ask for help. That help can be getting equipment ready, aid in holding the head or neck in position, or asking someone else to intubate. When faced with a difficult intubation you should call for backup, if such backup exists. Backup can be an anesthesiologist, any other intubator, or a surgeon to perform a possible tracheostomy. Safeguarding the patient is the first priority, and time is frequently of the essence.

Further Reading

Barrett GE, Coulthard SW: Upper airway obstruction: diagnosis and management options. *Anesthesia and ENT Surgery. Cont. Anesth. Pract.* 1987; 9: 73

Block C, Brechner VL: Unusual problems in airway management: II The influence of the temporomandibular joint, the mandible, and associated structures in endotracheal intubation. *Anesth. Analg.* 1971; 50: 114

Brechner VL: Unusual problems in airway management: I. Flexion, extension mobility of the cervical vertebrae. *Anesth. Analg.* 1968; 47: 362

Davies OD: Re-anesthetizing cases of tonsillectomy and adenoidectomy because of persistent postoperative hemorrhage. *Br. J. Anaes.* 1964; 36: 244

Donlon JV: Anesthetic management of the patient with compromised airways. *Anesth. Rev.* 1980; 7: 22

Gordon RA: Anesthetic management of patients with airway problems. *Int. Anesthesiol. Clin.* 1972; 10: 37

9

Nasal Intubation Techniques

N asal intubation is a useful technique to learn because it's sometimes the only safe way to intubate the patient.

Indications and Contraindications

You may prefer a nasal intubation for:

1. ease of patient positioning — placed awake so the patient can turn himself prone, etc.

2. long-term intubation, as in the ICU — nasal tubes are better tolerated, less tube movement

3. surgical access — nasal placement avoids surgical site in oral surgery, some facial fractures

4. minimize risk of aspiration — awake placement when there is risk of emesis, GI bleeding, bowel obstruction

5. difficult airway — awake intubation for short neck, morbid obesity, congenital anomaly, fractured mandible, inability to open mouth or move neck.

6. unstable cervical spine — awake intubation to identify symptoms during intubation, document neurologic status after intubation, avoid extension of neck during intubation

7. unstable hemodynamic status — awake for ICU or CCU patients in shock to avoid the risk of hypotension due to general anesthesia or sedation

We use nasal intubation frequently for emergency intubations in patients who are hemodynamically unstable, at risk for aspiration, or with anticipated difficult airways. You can perform awake oral intubations in all of the above situations. However, nasal intubations are often easier to perform and more comfortable for the awake patient than oral intubations.

Nasal intubations are contraindicated in patients with nasal fractures or basilar skull fractures. The risk of causing more damage or of intubating the brain through a fractured ethmoid sinus is too high. They are relatively contraindicated with a history of nose bleeds and sinusitis. Unavoidable inflamation and edema from the tube can cause a recurrence of bleeding and infection.

Techniques

Successful awake nasal intubations also start with assessment of the anatomy. To detect obstruction, pinch off each nostril in turn and then feel the amount of air exhaled through the other. Look for septal deviation. Avoid the effected side of the nose if there is a history of nose bleeds and sinusitis.

You can perform nasal intubations with the patient either awake or asleep. For awake placement the patient must breath spontaneously.

The best position for the head is still the sniffing position. Use a bit more flexion than extension. Extreme extension makes the angle that the tube must turn to enter the trachea more acute.

You must first anesthetize the nose. Several methods exist. To quickly numb the nose, combine one cc of one percent neosinephrine with four cc of viscous lidocaine. Dribble the mixture down the nares while the patient sniffs. Allow several minutes for the medication to work. You can also use five percent cocaine liquid or Afrin spray followed by lidocaine liquid. The secret is to use a combination that not only numbs but vasoconstricts. Neosinephrine or Afrin are added because all local anesthetics, except cocaine, cause vasodilation. Vasodilation produces edema, narrows the opening, and makes nosebleeds more likely. Thus, vasoconstrictors aid tube passage and minimize bleeding. Nasal topicalization can be accompanied by nerve block of the glossopharyngeal or superior laryngeal nerves as desired.

I frequently pass progressively larger nasal airways coated with local anesthetic ointment. I personally don't believe that this practice further dilates the nasal passage. However, this practice enhances the numbing. It also tests the passage for size and evidence of obstruction. Meanwhile, the patient becomes accustomed to the passage of nasal tubes, making passage of the larger endotracheal tube more tolerable.

Warming the tube in hot water makes it more pliable and easier to pass. Coat the tip of the tube with local anesthetic ointment. Gently slide it *straight back* into the nose, parallel to the floor of the nose (Fig. 9-1a). Avoid the common tendency to thread the tube into the frontal sinus, a painful maneuver likely to cause a nosebleed. Advance the tube until you feel a give or loss of resistance; the tube has just turned the corner into the posterior pharynx (Fig. 9-1b). Now slowly advance the tube during the patient's inspiration. Listen to the breath sounds through the tube. As long as the tube and the trachea are aligned you will hear hollow, loud breath sounds and see condensation inside the tube. Continue to advance the tube. If you run out of tube and still hear breath sounds you are in the trachea (Fig. 9-1c). Successful placement often makes the patient cough.

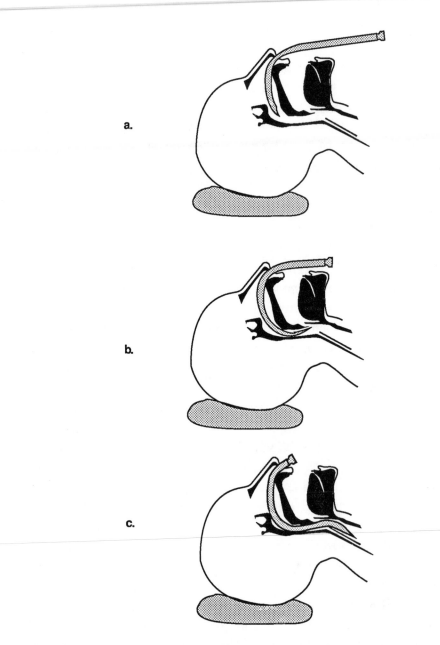

Fig. 9-1. Technique of blind nasal intubation.

Check immediately that you have really intubated the patient. Inflate the cuff and check for the presence of bilateral breath sounds. With the patient breathing spontaneously, you will feel the air moving in and out of the tube. When she ventilates spontaneously you'll feel the bag collapse with each breath. She won't be able to speak once the tube passes between the cords. Condensation will form inside the tube as she breathes. When you ventilate the patient the chest rises as you squeeze the bag.

Make sure that the breath sounds are bilateral and equal. If there is a mainstem intubation slowly pull the tube back until bilateral breath sounds reappear.

I believe that the cuff should always be inflated once the patient is intubated. Sometimes people leave the cuff deflated so that the patient can talk around the tube. I believe that this risks aspiration. The tube holds the cords apart and defeats the normal protective mechanisms. Secretions can dribble down the outside of the tube into the trachea.

If the tube passes into the esophagus, breath sounds vanish. The patient frequently gags. Stop, pull the tube back until you hear breath sounds again, then slowly advance once more. If the tube tip catches in the vallecula or one of the piriform sinuses, you'll hear good breath sounds but won't be able to pass the tube. Try gently twisting the tube a bit as you advance. Also try flexing or extending the head. Both maneuvers change the angle of the endotracheal tube and frequently let the tip slide off the obstruction and into the trachea.

If you can't hear breath sounds once the tube has entered the posterior pharynx or if you feel alot of resistance, stop advancing the tube. Check to make sure that the tube tip is not dissecting submucosally. This occurs when the tip tears the nasal lining and slides underneath. The patient often complains of severe pain when this happens. With submucosal dissection you won't see the tube in the posterior pharynx but you will see a bulge behind the tonsillar pillars. When the tube is submucosal, carefully remove it. Be prepared for a heavy nosebleed. If nasal intubation is still indicated try the other nares and proceed carefully.

You may need to consider postponing elective surgery because of the risk of retropharyngeal hematoma and abscess formation.

If the tube won't enter the trachea easily, turn the head toward the side or change the degree of flexion or extension (Fig. 9-2a-c). If

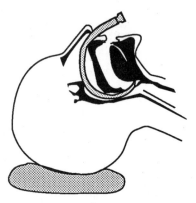

a. ENDOTRACHEAL TUBE CAUGHT IN THE VALLECULA

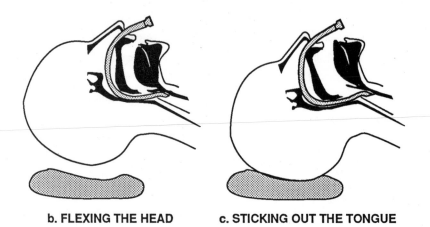

b. FLEXING THE HEAD   **c. STICKING OUT THE TONGUE**

Fig. 9-2. If the tube tip stops in the valecula, or the piriform sinus, flex the head slightly or have the patient open her mouth and stick her tongue out. Both change the angle of the tube.

movement in one direction doesn't work, turn it the other way. Picture where you're aiming the tip of the tube and adjust the head accordingly. A tube placed in the right nostril tends to cross to the left lower pharynx. Therefore moving the head slightly to the right of midline for a right sided tube will align the trachea with the tube. For left nasal intubations move the head to the left. Pushing the larynx toward the side opposite the nares being used can also help.

Sometimes further topicalization or sedation will smooth the intubation. However, you must weigh the risks of these maneuvers against the benefits. An overly sedated patient with a numb larynx can aspirate rather easily.

When the tube won't pass blindly, you can use your laryngoscope to visualize the larynx (Fig. 9-3). I usually use a Mac blade for this maneuver. It gives me more room to manipulate the tube. Once you see the larynx hold your left hand firmly in position. Have an assistant push the tube into the trachea while you guide the tip of the tube with magill forceps or some other instrument. Never grab the cuff of

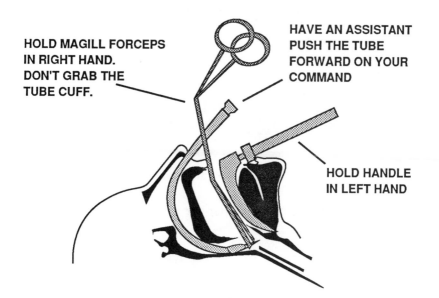

HOLD MAGILL FORCEPS
IN RIGHT HAND.
DON'T GRAB THE
TUBE CUFF.

HAVE AN ASSISTANT
PUSH THE TUBE
FORWARD ON YOUR
COMMAND

HOLD HANDLE
IN LEFT HAND

Fig. 9-3. Using the Magill forceps to intubate.

the tube with your forceps. You can easily rip it, leaving no way to seal off the trachea. You can use this useful technique on either awake or anesthetized patients. The patient can also be apneic during placement under direct visualization. You can use a bent stylet or a hook to curve the endotracheal tube anteriorly if you don't have Magill forceps.

Often the endotracheal tube aims at the larynx but won't enter. A firm catheter passed through the endotracheal tube when it's lined up may enter the trachea and provide a guide to insert the tube. Nasogastric tubes or tube exchangers are useful for this purpose. Firmly hold the endotracheal tube at the point where breath sounds are most audible, then pass the catheter through the tube. Slide the tube over the catheter into the larynx. Check breath sounds (Fig. 9-4).

One final caveat with the combined oral/ nasal technique. Sometimes you can't see the trachea. If the patient is breathing, listen for breath sounds as you pass the tube. By using their loudness to guide your aim you can blindly intubate a patient during direct laryngoscopy.

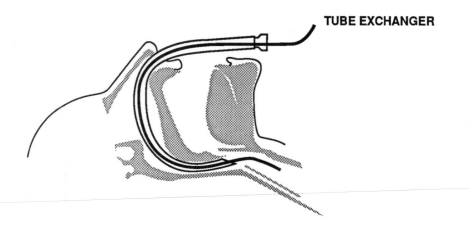

TUBE EXCHANGER

Fig. 9-4. Using a tube exchanger to assist intubation.

Further Reading

Pederson B: Blind nasotracheal intubation: A review and a new guided technique. *Acta. Anaesth. Scandinav.* 1971; 15: 107

10

Management of the Airway — Establishing an Airway

O pening an obstructed airway is a different skill from intubation, but the two are inseparable. The ability to ventilate a patient is often more important than the ability to intubate a patient. Intubation is merely one means of ventilating and protecting the airway. Rarely will intubation, itself, save a life. Ventilation, on the other hand, frequently saves lives.

If the patient is apneic proceed immediately to ventilate him or her with a bag and a mask. On the other hand, if the patient is breathing spontaneously, but is obstructed, there are several ways to open the airway.

The easiest is to grab the mandible behind each jaw angle and lift. Also, extend the head if there is no risk of cervical spine injury. Both maneuvers pull the tongue and associated structures upward and usually relieve the obstruction (Fig. 10-1a-d, 10-2a, b). Because pressing on the angle of the jaw is painful, this maneuver often has the benefit of waking a stuporous patient — another means of improving the airway.

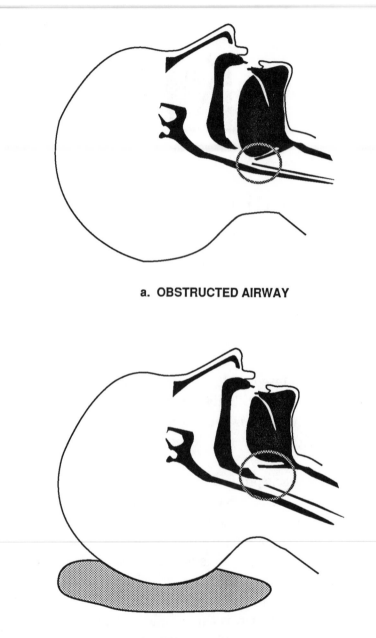

a. OBSTRUCTED AIRWAY

b. SNIFFING POSITION

Fig. 10-1a, b. Opening an obstructed airway. (See following page for continuation.)

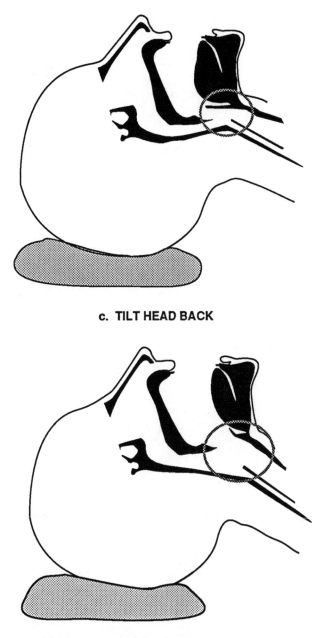

c. TILT HEAD BACK

d. PULL THE ANGLES OF THE JAW UPWARD

Fig. 10-1c, d. Opening an obstructed airway.

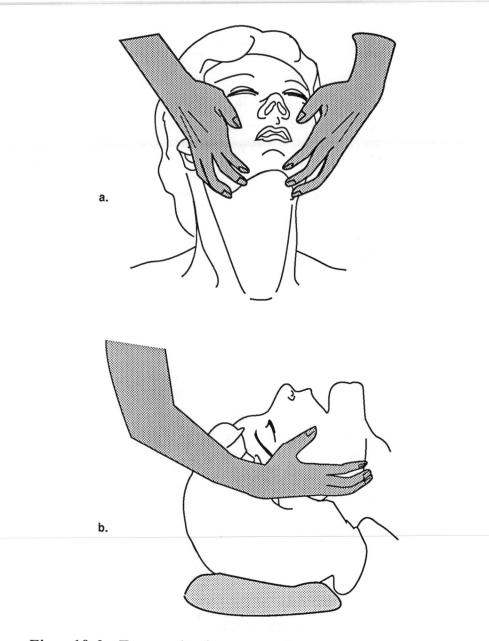

a.

b.

Fig. 10-2. To open the airway, extend the head and thrust the jaw
forward.

If you still have a marginal airway insert a nasal or an oral airway. See Table 10-1 for the signs of airway obstruction.

Terminology can sometimes be confusing. Not only do we call the patient's passageway from mouth to trachea his airway, we also call the tools to establish an open breathing passage airways as well. Context usually makes the meaning clear.

Table 10-1. Evidence of Airway Obstruction

- stridor

- poor movement of air

- faint or absent breath sounds

- use of accessory muscles of respiration

- rocking chest motion:
  chest falls on inspiration\
  abdomen rises on inspiration

- cyanosis

Use of the Nasal Airway

Nasal airways are soft, flexible tubes which slide through one side of the nose. This positions the opening of the tube in the posterior pharynx, behind the tongue. The opening is often, though not always, in line with the trachea.

Awake patients often tolerate a nasal airway better than an oral airway because it stimulates the gag reflex less. Liberally coat your nasal airway with some lubricating ointment if available. Local anesthetic ointment has the advantage of numbing the nose and making the tube more easily tolerated. However, water or non-anesthetic jelly works as well. Slide the nasal airway into the nares and gently advance it along the *floor* of the nose (Fig. 10-3a, b). The beginner will frequently try

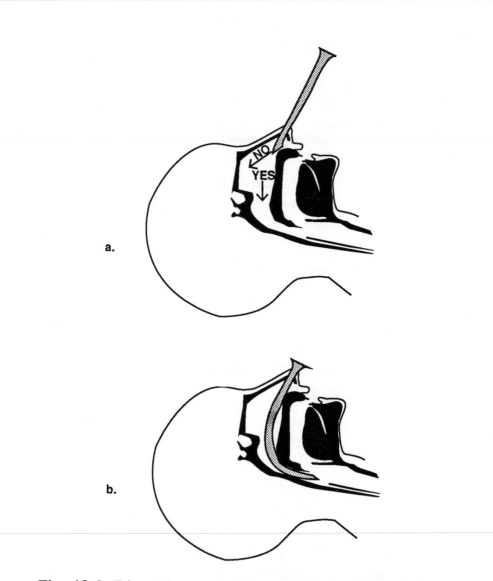

Fig. 10-3. Direct the nasal airway along the floor of the nose. Slide it forward to position it in the posterior pharynx.

to thread the nasal airway up the nose toward the frontal sinus. Not only will the tube not pass in this direction, you risk a nose bleed. If you meet an obstruction then carefully twist the tube while slowly pushing it forward. Don't force it. Check your angle of insertion and try again. If the nasal airway will not pass, try the other nares or switch to a smaller tube.

The nasal passage sometimes pinches the tube as it turns the corner. This may make suctioning down the nasal airway difficult because the narrowing may prevent passage of a suction catheter.

You can use a nasal airway to ventilate any patient when ventilation with a bag and a mask are difficult. Simply insert an endotracheal tube connector into the nasal end of a nasal airway. Choose one that fits snugly. The nasal airway will now connect to your ventilation circuit. Hold the mouth and the opposite nostril firmly closed. Squeezing the bag will now ventilate the patient (Fig. 10-4).

Use of the Oral Airway

An oral airway is a fairly firm, curved piece of plastic. It sits on top of the tongue and pulls the tongue and associated structures forward. Oral airways have several disadvantages.

First, the oral airway must be placed inside the mouth between the patient's teeth, sometimes a difficult and personally risky task in an awake patient who is protecting her airway. Never place your unprotected fingers inside a patient's mouth unless you're fairly certain that he or she can't bite you. Fortunately, there are several ways of inserting oral airways without having to so this.

Second, firm, plastic oral airways can damage teeth — especially if the teeth are already loose or decayed.

Third, the tip of the oral airway sits on the back of the tongue. An awake patient will sometimes gag, vomit and possibly aspirate. This is especially true if the patient's mental status is compromised.

Having stated the disadvantages, let me also state that oral airways

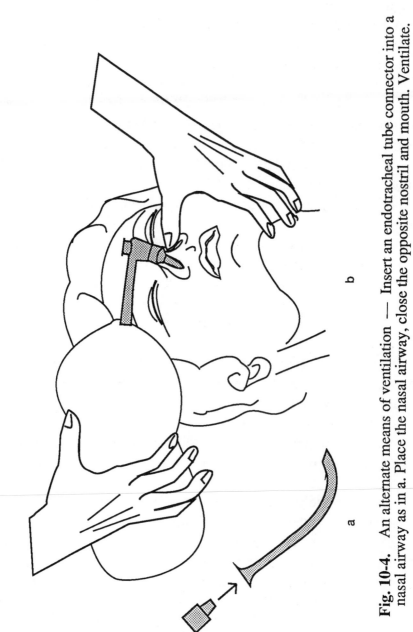
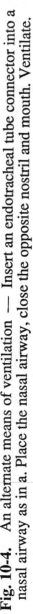

Fig. 10-4. An alternate means of ventilation — Insert an endotracheal tube connector into a nasal airway as in a. Place the nasal airway, close the opposite nostril and mouth. Ventilate.

relieve most types of obstruction very effectively. They are one of our most important tools. The correct size oral airway places the flange immediately outside the teeth or gums and positions the tip near the vallecula. To estimate the correct size, place the airway next to the patient's jaw parallel to the mouth and judge where it will lie. Too small an airway places the tip in the middle of the tongue. This bunches the tissue and worsens obstruction. Too large an airway will extend from the mouth and prevent sealing the mask over the face.

There are several ways to insert an oral airway. Open the mouth widely, as you would to intubate the patient. Insert the oral airway with the curve either down toward the tongue, or up toward the roof of the mouth. With the curve down, advance the airway until the tip is behind the back of the tongue. Properly placed the airway pulls the tongue forward. Improperly placed it pushes the tongue into the back of the pharynx and further obstructs the airway. Wetting the airway with water will allow it to slide more easily.

You can use a tongue blade in the left hand to help open the mouth and push the tongue down. Place the tongue blade to the rear of the tongue and pull it forward. Often this allows you to slide the oral airway in without any further problem (10-5a, b). At this point, if I still can't insert the airway, I grasp it firmly in my right hand and force it to straighten as much as possible (Fig. 10-6a, b). I then place the straightened airway on the tongue blade and slide it down the blade to the back of the mouth. Once in position I relax my grip. The oral airway springs back into its curve and pulls the tongue forward.

Many people insert an oral airway by turning its curve toward the roof of the mouth. They advance it until its tip lies behind the tongue and then flip the airway into position (Fig. 10-7a, b). While very effective, you must use caution. You can easily damage teeth and the roof of the mouth, especially if the mouth is not wide open.

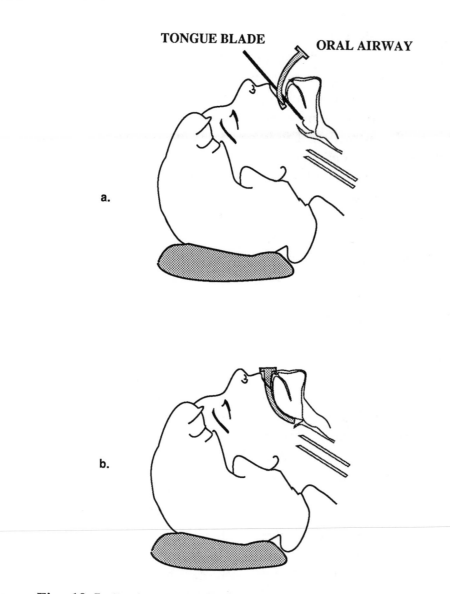

TONGUE BLADE   **ORAL AIRWAY**

a.

b.

Fig. 10-5. Push tongue down with tongue blade, then slide the oral airway into positon.

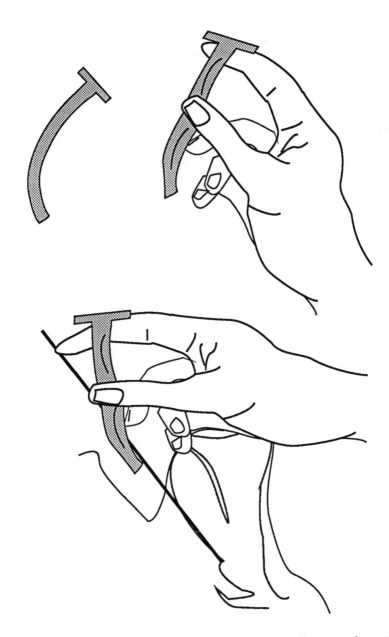

Fig. 10-6. Straighten the oral airway with your fingers, then slide it down the tongue blade until the tip is behind the tongue.

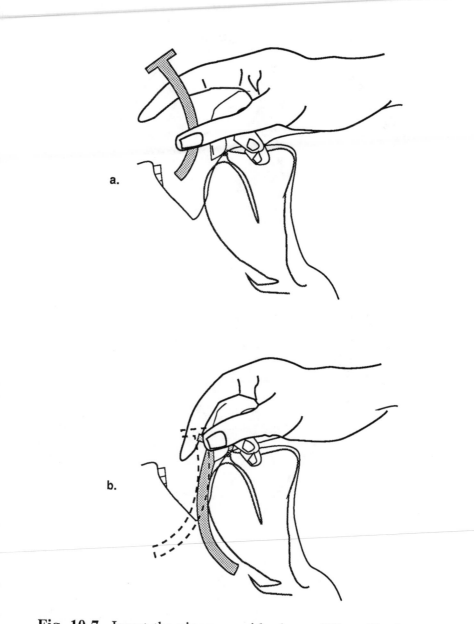

Fig. 10-7. Insert the airway upside down. When flipping the airway, make sure that you avoid pressure on the upper teeth. The hard plastic can also scrape the roof of the mouth.

Ventilating With a Bag and a Mask

Having established the airway you should next check ventilation. If the patient is breathing adequately, you can decide the need for intubation and for such treatments as narcotic reversal with less haste. Apply oxygen by mask while you do this. If the patient is not breathing well you must immediately assist or control his respiration. Both require the use of some form of bag and mask apparatus.

For the bag and mask to work you must have a good seal on the mask. This means pressing the mask against the patient's face to effectively prevent the escape of the pressurized breaths you deliver.

First, choose the correct size mask for the patient. Most women take a small mask. Most men will use a medium. Tall men may need a large. Large children need a 3, toddlers a 2, infants a 1. The proper size just covers the space between the bridge of the nose and the crease in the chin. The entire upper and lower lips fit inside the mask. If you choose too small or too large a mask, you may find it hard to get a good seal.

Pull the head into extension and open the airway (Fig. 10-8a). Hold it there with your left hand. All masks are triangular in shape. Place the apex of the triangle on the bridge of the nose and press firmly (Fig. 10-8b). Grasp each side of the mask with your hands and spread as much as you can. This is easier with some masks than others. As you spread, reach down with your free index and middle fingers and pull the loose cheek tissue forward to bunch on either side of the mouth. Place your remaining fingers on the jaw bone and pull upward. This action also holds the head in extension and holds the airway open while you position the mask. Now, lower the mask over the cheeks and allow the edges to grab the bunched cheek tissue (Fig. 10-8c, d). Make sure the lower lip is inside the mask. Take your right hand off the mask and maintain your seal and jaw lift with the left (Fig. 10-9). Squeeze the bag with your right hand. If you have a good seal no air will escape around the mask. You can tolerate some leak as long as you can ventilate the patient. If not, you must get a better fit.

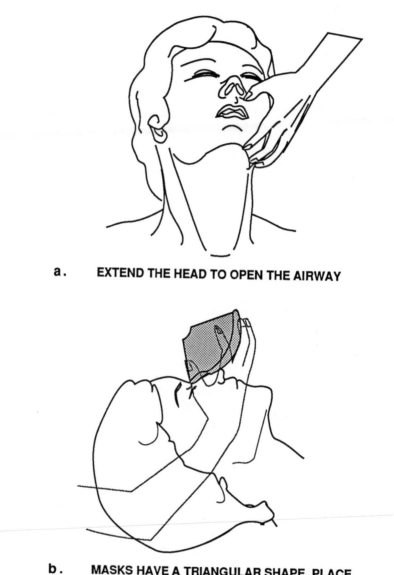

a. EXTEND THE HEAD TO OPEN THE AIRWAY

b. MASKS HAVE A TRIANGULAR SHAPE. PLACE THE APEX OF THE TRIANGLE OVER THE BRIDGE OF THE NOSE.

Fig. 10-8a, b. Getting a good mask seal. (See following page for continuation.)

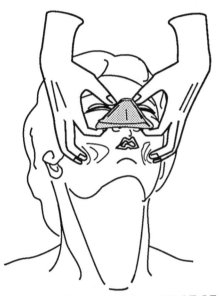

c . **HOLD MASK TOP AGAINST BRIDGE OF NOSE.
SPREAD SIDES WITH HANDS. PUSH CHEEK
TISSUE UNDER MASK EDGES.**

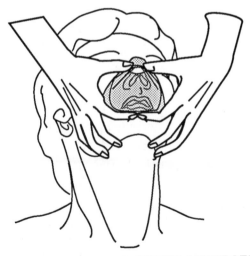

d . **LOWER MASK OVER CHEEKS. LET EDGES GRAB
BUNCHED TISSUE. SEAT OVER CHIN. MAKE SURE
LOWER LIP IS INSIDE MASK.**

Fig. 10-8c, d. Getting a good mask seal.

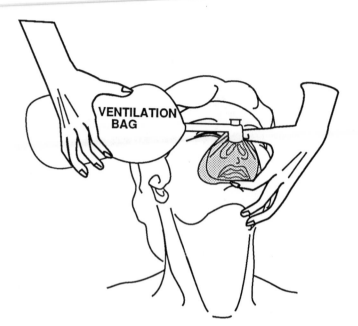

Fig. 10-9. Holding the mask while squeezing the bag.

The extra bulk of the bunched cheek tissue fills in the gaps between the mask and the patient and helps seal it. In certain patient's, especially edentulous ones, this may not work. Typically the mask leaks on the side opposite the hand holding the mask. First, use the weight of the bag on the leaky side to force the mask against the patient's face. If this doesn't work, then place gauze in the gap to seal the hole. Alternatively, you can ask a helper to push the cheek up against the outside of the mask at the leak sites. This seals the hole very effectively. Once again use your helpers if you have problems.

Large, edentulous, or fat patients occasionally force you to use both hands to seal the mask. In this situation, place one hand on either side of the mask (Fig. 10-10). Place your thumbs at the top of the mask and hold the bottom of the mask down forcefully with your index fingers. Pull the jaw upward with your remaining fingers by spreading them along the jaw line. Hold just the bone. Pushing on the soft tissue under the jaw can force it into the airway and worsen obstruction. The

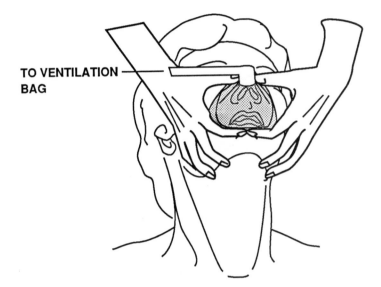

Fig. 10-10. Using both hands to seal the mask.

basic hand position is the same as that just described. You just leave both hands on the mask and have an assistant ventilate the patient. Move your fingers as needed to perfect your seal. Even when using both hands on the mask, you may need a helper to stop the leaks.

The ability to ventilate is the ultimate test of success in positioning both patient and equipment. Squeeze the bag. The chest should rise with each breath. Have a helper listen to the chest to verify breath sounds as you ventilate. As you squeeze the bag pay attention to the resistance you feel as the lungs inflate. Obstruction makes squeezing the bag difficult or impossible. A leak in the ventilation system makes squeezing the bag extremely easy. In both these cases, however, the chest won't rise. Educating your hand is valuable because it allows you to monitor your patient without staring at the chest. If you can tell how well you ventilate the patient without looking you free your attention for other matters. Don't forget that difficulty in ventilation may be due to your patient's illness and not to your technique. Congestive heart failure, bronchospasm, and pneumothorax can also make airway resistance worse, breath sounds fainter, and ventilation difficult. You must prove, however, that the fault is not your own before blaming poor ventilation on the patient.

Placing oral or nasal airways at this point may improve your ventilation if you have not already done so. Suction the secretions, if any, to prevent aspiration.

In my opinion, the ability to handle airway obstruction and to ventilate with a bag and a mask are equally as important, if not more important, than the ability to intubate. Practice at every available opportunity.

Needle Cricothyroidotomy

Needle cricothyroidotomy is a fast, easy way of providing oxygen to a patient with an obstructed airway who does not respond to the previous steps. It will buy you time to establish a more permanent airway such as an intubation or a tracheostomy if the patient is hypoxic.

First, identify the cricothyroid membrane by finding the cricoid ring. The membrane lies in the gap between the ring and the thyroid cartilage above it (Fig. 10-11). You can use any intravenous catheter-over-needle set to puncture the cricothyroid membrane. Attach a syringe to the hub of the needle and aspirate as you advance. The aspiration of air verifies intra-tracheal placement. Slide the catheter off the needle into the trachea. Again attach your syringe to the hub of the catheter and aspirate air to check placement. Use the largest intravenous catheter available, such as a size 10 or 14 gauge.

You now need to connect the catheter to a ventilation system. Because of its small diameter, the best means of giving oxygen through this device is a jet ventilator. Unfortunately, this sophisticated piece of equipment is rarely present when you need it.

The connector from a number 3 endotracheal tube fits snugly into the hub of any intravenous catheter. The catheter will now connect to your ventilation bag. However, this tiny assembly is often difficult to hold while you're squeezing the bag. I prefer to place the connector from a number 7.5 endotracheal tube into the barrel of a 3 cc syringe. The barrel of your syringe now mates to the hub of your catheter and gives you something more substantial to hold. You must ventilate vigorously to pass enough oxygen through the catheter. Gas will passively escape from the mouth.

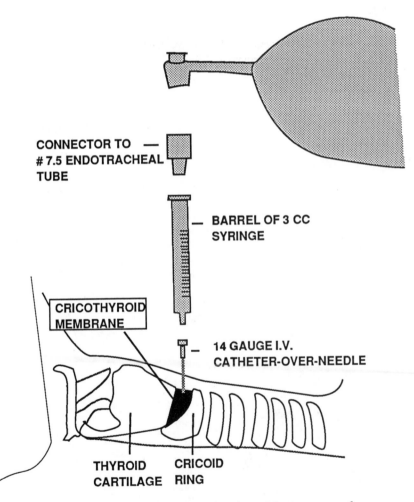

CONNECTOR TO —
 # 7.5 ENDOTRACHEAL
TUBE

— BARREL OF 3 CC
SYRINGE

CRICOTHYROID
MEMBRANE

— 14 GAUGE I.V.
CATHETER-OVER-NEEDLE

THYROID   CRICOID
CARTILAGE   RING

Fig. 10-11. Emergency needle cricothyroidostomy and a means of connecting it to a ventilation system.

Reports indicate that patients can maintain themselves for several minutes breathing spontaneously through an 10g catheter. If you use a 14-16g catheter you often need high pressure oxygen for adequate ventilation. However, any oxygen supplied during emergency treatment of airway obstruction is useful.

Surgical cricothyroidotomy is described in Chapter 12.

Further Reading

Lopez NR: Mechanical problems of the airway. *Clin. Anes.* 1968; 3: 8
Linscott MS, Horton WC: Management of upper airway obstruction. *Otolaryngol. Clin. North Am.* 1979; 12:351-373

11

Complications

A ny technique that we learn in medicine has potential complications. Fortunately, most complications are uncommon. Understanding the causes and routinely taking the steps to prevent them will ensure that they stay uncommon.

Complications from intubation can occur at any time — during the intubation procedure, while the patient remains intubated, or following the extubation (Table 11-1).

Complications Occurring During the Intubation

Mechanical technique and the response of the patient cause the main problems that arise during the intubation. Trauma from excessive force or improper use of the laryngoscope blade can cause edema, bleeding, and damage to the teeth and soft tissue. Trauma frequently occurs in

Table 11-1. Complications of Tracheal Intubation

DURING INTUBATION

Mechanical
trauma to teeth and soft tissue
tube damage requiring change
esophageal intubation
submucosal dissection
bleeding in the oropharynx, nose

Physiologic Response of Patient
hypertension
arrhythmia, including tachycardia
aspiration
hypoxia
hypercarbia and acidosis
CPR interrupted > 15 seconds
pneumothorax caused or worsened
laryngospasm
bronchospasm

WHILE INTUBATED

tube obstruction: secretions, blood, biting tube, kinking
mainstem intubation
esophageal intubation
accidental extubation
mucosal ischemia: excessive cuff pressure, tube tip
higher resistance to breathing
aspiration around cuff or tube
pneumonia
sinusitis (with nasal intubation)

AFTER EXTUBATION

Acute
laryngospasm
vomiting and aspiration
sore throat
hoarseness
laryngeal edema, subglottic edema

Chronic
mucosal ulceration
tracheitis
tracheal stenosis
vocal cord paralysis
arytenoid cartilage dislocation

---

emergency situations when the intubator must hurry. Positioning is often less than optimal. Struggling in the conscious patient can prolong intubation attempts. The presence of a difficult airway also prolongs intubation.

Prolonged intubations predispose to the harmful physiologic responses of the patient listed in Table 11-1. Hypertension, arrhythmia, hypoxia, hypercapnia and respiratory acidosis, vomiting, and aspiration can all occur. Laryngospasm and bronchospasm from airway irritability or aspirated secretions happen more frequently. The intubator tends to become so fixated on the intubation that he or she forgets the patient. The temptation to interrupt CPR for longer than 15 seconds is great. It's also easy to forget to ventilate the patient between attempts and to suction the mouth.

The first step in preventing these complications is to place the care of the patient above the intubation itself. As long as you can ventilate the patient you have the time

- to do a gentle, purposeful intubation,

- to alter your technique and equipment,

- to reposition the patient, and

- to call for assistance.

You can *cautiously* sedate awake patients in the emergency situation — *being careful to avoid the loss of their respiratory drive or loss of their airway.* Treat hypertension and arrhythmia. Oxygenate and ventilate the patient between attempts. If you can't ventilate the patient then you shouldn't spend a long time on an intubation attempt.

Attention to the patient will slow you down a little bit. It will also keep your patient healthier. Because you're taking more time you will be less likely to traumatize.

Patients with irritable bronchi such as asthmatics or those with chronic obstructive pulmonary disease often develop bronchospasm, or wheezing. Topicalization of the trachea with 1% lidocaine — i.e., cardiac lidocaine 3-5 cc sprayed down the tube — may improve the patient's tolerance to the tube. The most common cause of wheezing in an intubated patient, however, is an endotracheal tube tip that either touches the carina or enters a bronchus. When you hear wheezing, check the depth of insertion and listen for the equality of breath sounds. Breath sounds may be equal if the tip is merely touching the carina. Try pulling the tube back slightly to see if this makes a difference. If the wheezing disappears you have your diagnosis. If it doesn't, treat the bronchospasm and get an X-ray as soon as you can.

If your patient vomits during the intubation attempt turn her on her side and quickly suction the pharynx. Place the bed in Trendelenburg if you can. Fast action can often prevent aspiration. Proceed with the intubation and immediately suction the endotracheal tube after you've placed it. Verify breath sounds. Wheezing, unequal breath sounds, an acidic pH. of the tracheal secretions, or actual vomitus or particulate matter in the endotracheal tube indicate a major aspiration. Aspirating as little as 0.4 ml/kg of pH 2.5 liquid can cause severe pneumonitis. Minor aspiration may remain asymptomatic. Treat major aspiration aggressively with bronchoscopy, tracheal toilet, and chest physiotherapy.

If the patient aspirates upon extubation you must use your clinical judgement as to the necessity of reintubation. Extubated patients are much better able to cough and deep breathe than intubated patients. On the other hand, applying positive inspiratory pressure or high concentrations of oxygen is much easier in the intubated patient. Let the patient's status be your guide.

Complications Occurring While Intubated

Mechanical problems with the endotracheal tube cause most of the complications during the period of intubation.

Patient movement will move the endotracheal tube. The tip of the tube follows the nose. If the nose points up, the tube rises in the larynx. If the nose points down, the tube descends. Extubation, esophageal intubation, and mainstem intubation can occur at any time. Nasal intubations minimize ascent or descent and thus are often preferred for long-standing intubations. Loose taping of the tube allows excessive movement.

Trauma to the trachea is the other major problem with movement of the tube. In fact, twisting of the tube can force its tip against the mucosa and cause ulceration. Secure the tube well to minimize the risk of trauma and misplacement. Avoid unnecessary patient movement. Use supports to prevent twisting of the tube.

Excessive inflation of the tube cuff also causes mucosal damage. Inflation to "minimal seal" and the use of pressure measuring devices can minimize this. Normally we inflate cuffs to 15 mmHg. This pressure usually prevents aspiration but is below the critical 25 mmHg pressure when mucosal ischemia starts to occur. Using the largest tube possible minimizes the cuff pressure needed to seal the trachea. This reduces the gap that the cuff must seal and therefore lowers the volume and pressure needed to do so. The cuff on the larger tube spreads the

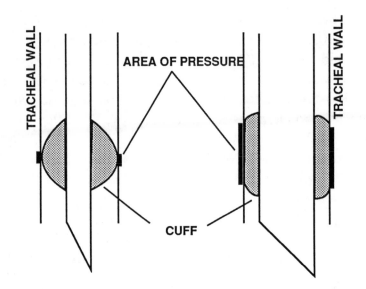

Fig. 11-1. Demonstration of cuff pressure distribution with different sized tubes. The wider the area of spread, the lower the pressure per square mm.

pressure more equally over the tracheal wall. The cuff on the smaller tube becomes rounded when distended and applies point pressure to the wall (Fig. 11-1).

Breathing through an endotracheal requires more force because the resistance is higher. This resistance increases in direct proportion to the length of the tube and to the *fourth* power of the radius of the tube. It makes sense that using the largest diameter tube will decrease this resistance. Weaning a respiratory cripple from a ventilator may depend on such small advantages.

Larger tubes also make the risk of obstruction less. They are far less likely to kink or plug with dried secretions or blood. Meticulous attention to tube positioning and cleansing of the tube will also prevent such dangerous obstructions. Allowing the patient to bite on the tube will also cause obstruction on occasion.

A final problem comes from infection. The larynx is a major barrier to infection. The endotracheal tube violates this barrier.

Although sterile at the start of intubation, the endotracheal tube must pass through the mouth to enter the trachea. Bacteria can enter the lungs. Patients intubated for prolonged periods often have poorer oral hygiene. It's hard to brush your teeth with an endotracheal tube in place. Secretions passing the cuff and poor technique in suctioning the patient also allow bacteria to enter. In addition, intubated patients cough poorly. They can't close their glottis to generate the higher pressures needed to cough. Pneumonia can occur. Edema from minor tube trauma can cause obstruction of the sinuses and eustachian tubes, especially with nasal intubations. This predisposes to ear and sinus infections. Close attention to oral hygiene, careful asepsis, and frequent examination of the patient will help prevent infection.

Complications Following Extubation

Acute and chronic problems can follow extubation.

Laryngospasm usually occurs when the patient is only partially conscious at the moment of extubation. Extubation when the patient is still in stage 2 anesthesia, the excitement stage, is one example. In anesthesia we try to extubate patients either deeply anesthetized or totally awake — never in stage 2. At this time secretions or stimulation of the vocal cords causes reflex protective spasm. Unfortunately the rest of the brain is too asleep to turn it off. The patient may become hypoxic. Patients suffering from head trauma or heavy sedation are also at risk.

Treat laryngospasm with oxygen, positive pressure, and forceful upward pull on the jaw. Intravenous lidocaine 0.5-1 mg/kg sometimes helps. Only use muscle relaxants if you are experienced in their use. You can avoid laryngospasm by never extubating your patient partially awake, by carefully suctioning any secretions before extubation, and by being gentle.

Vomiting and aspiration can occur. Prepare for this with suction and heightened vigilance.

Minor edema often causes sore throats and hoarseness. Major

edema causes airway obstruction. Young age predisposes the patient to problems simply because the small size of their airway makes even minor edema more important. Other predispositions include using too large a tube in a child, traumatic intubation, airway infection, and prolonged intubation. Tube trauma from excessive tube movement or an overinflated cuff can also cause problems.

Major edema of the larynx presents as post extubation croup. The patient, typically a child, develops a barking cough. The patient may have stridor or dyspnea. Conservative therapy consists of humidified oxygen by mask or a "croup tent" or treatment with aerosolized racemic epinephrine. This often shrinks the mucous membranes and resolves the obstruction. The dose of racemic epinephrine is 0.25 - 0.5 cc of 2.25% solution in 5 cc saline every 1-4 hours depending on the severity. Dexamethasone, 0.15 mg/kg may help prevent further edema formation. Severe cases may need reintubation. Croup can develop as long as 1-2 hours following extubation.

Tracheitis, tracheal stenosis, vocal cord paralysis, arytenoid cartilage dislocation all represent chronic complications. You can minimize the risk of the problems by the use of gentle technique and care throughout the patients intubation.

It is far better to prevent complications than to show skill in treating them. Forewarned is forearmed.

Further Reading

Byrum LJ, Pierce AK: Pulmonary aspiration of gastric contents. *Am. Rev. Respir. Dis.* 1976; 114: 1129

Harley HR: Laryngotracheal obstruction complicating tracheostomy or endotracheal intubation with assisted respiration. A Critical Review. *Thorax* 1971; 26: 493

Knowleson GTG, Bennett HFM: The pressures exerted on the trachea by endotracheal inflatable cuffs. *Br. J. Anaes.* 1970; 42: 834

Tarle DA, Chandler JE, Good JT, et.al.: Emergency room intubation — Complications and survival. *Chest* 1979; 75: 541

Vandam LD: Vomiting of gastric contents during the operative period. *N. Eng. J. Med.* 1965; 273: 1206

12

Specialized Equipment

U p until now we've discussed intubation using the standard equipment readily available in operating rooms, emergency rooms, ambulances, and cardiac arrest carts. Anesthesiologists, intensive care specialists, and surgeons occasionally use more specialized equipment to intubate patients with difficult airways. You usually won't find this equipment in the emergency room or on the ward because you rarely need it. Its expense, fragility, and increased risk of complication make it less suitable for those not trained in its use. Knowledge of its existence, however, will alert you to potential solutions to difficult airway problems.

Safeguarding Your Patient's Safety

It's easy to loose track of time when performing any of the following maneuvers. Therefore, use the following safety precautions.

Monitor the patient's oxygenation. Observe the patient's color. Use a pulse oximeter to measure the patient's oxygen saturation, if you have one. Keep the O_2 saturation above 90%, corresponding to a PO_2t above 60 mmHg. To tell you the exact PO_2 and PCO_2 and thus identify hypoventilation, hypercarbia, and hypoxemia you need arterial blood gases. However, these results often take more than 10-15 minutes to arrive even in a large hospital — sometimes too late to help in a crisis. Always provide extra oxygen when available.

Have your assistant time any period of apnea occurring during airway instrumentation. If it takes more than one or two minutes to perform any maneuver in the apneic patient, stop and ventilate. Let any awake patient "catch his breath" during a prolonged attempt. It helps him or her tolerate the procedure better and gives you a chance to gather your thoughts. Have an assistant monitor vital signs while you concentrate on the airway. High blood pressure and fast heart rates harm some patients as much as the lack of oxgen.

Tell the patient what you're doing. Be supportive. Cooperative patients make intubation safer and easier.

Suction the airway frequently. Gagging on the instruments can cause vomiting and even an alert patient can aspirate. After intubation, suction the endotracheal tube well.

Use sedation and local anesthesia judiciously, but watch for complications and overdose (see Chapter 13).

Discuss problems with more experienced intubators and ask for their advice and help. Asking for help during intubation should never threaten your ego. Asking for assistance only helps your patient.

Flexible Guides

Endotracheal tubes often enter the esophagus during difficult intubations because they don't curve enough to enter an anterior larynx. You can sometimes enter the larynx with an LTA, or laryngotracheal anesthesia kit, and then use it as a guide for threading the endotracheal tube. An LTA is simply a lidocaine-filled syringe attached to a long, stiff, curved catheter. It's normally used to squirt lidocaine down the trachea to prevent wheezing or hypertension during intubation. Place the LTA beside the endotracheal tube and insert it through the

Murphy eye *from the outside* (Fig. 12-1). Aim the catheter upward into the larynx and then slide the endotracheal tube over it and into the trachea. You can substitute a stylet for the LTA. Be very gentle in order to avoid damaging the trachea.

The Flexguide NCC (Fig. 12-2) consists of a barrel with a thumb ring plunger, attached to a long, thin rod about 6 cm (2.5 inches) longer than an endotracheal tube. Pushing the plunger curves the tip of the rod up. Insert the rod into your tube until the barrel seats into the 15 mm adapter, allowing them to act as a unit. Perform routine direct laryngoscopy and aim the tip of the rod into the larynx, maneuvering the tip as necessary. The Flexguide is often awkward to use because the right hand is at operator eye level. Keep your arm and back straight to minimize this problem. Standing on a stool helps.

Whenever you intubate without seeing the vocal cords, immediately check proper tube placement. Esophageal intubation easily occurs.

Manipulating Endotracheal Tubes, Blades and Handles

Nasal endotracheal tubes sometimes enter the esophagus because they won't curve forward enough after entering the oropharynx.

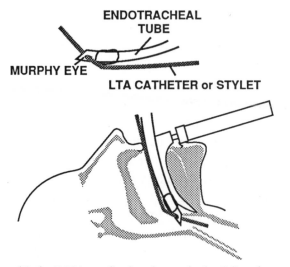

Fig. 12-1. LTA or Stylet through the Murphy eye.

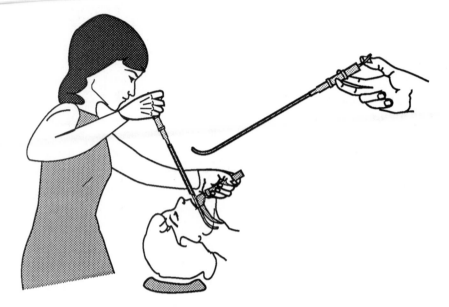

Fig. 12-2. Using the Flexguide.

Endotrol tubes solve this problem with a pull cord attached to a ring near the 15 mm adapter. Pulling the ring turns the tip of the tube anteriorly, allowing you to manipulate the tip with more precise control.

Having an assistant use a hook to pull the tip of the tube forward during nasal intubation also works (Fig. 12-3.)

Tube benders grab the tube *behind the cuff* and bend it upward when you close the jaws.

Many variations on laryngoscope blades and handles exist. The polio blade (Fig.12-4) was invented to intubate polio patients inside an "iron lung." Encasing the patient's body in a machine made conventional laryngoscopy difficult — you couldn't extend the head or position the handle over the chest. The polio blade is a straight blade which attaches to the handle at an angle of nearly 180°. Postioning the handle over the patient's head changes the angle of lift. You usually don't need to tilt the head to see the larynx, useful in neck-injured patients. Don't lever the blade against the upper teeth, lift the mandible away from you.

A Howland lock (Fig. 12-5) fits onto the top of the standard handle. It increases the angle of the blade, allowing you to lift the blade

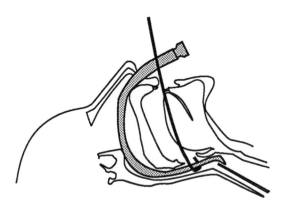

Fig. 12-3. Using a hook to help pass a tube with too little curvature.

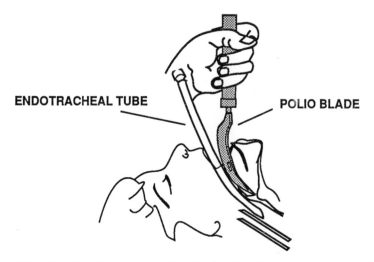

ENDOTRACHEAL TUBE   **POLIO BLADE**

Fig. 12-4. Using the polio blade. Don't press on the teeth.

more forcefully without levering on the teeth. The angulation of the lock makes it more awkward to use in a barrel-chested patient.

Some handles let you vary the angle of the blade from a sharp bend to complete extension, based on the clinical situation.

Huffman Prisms attach to the MacIntosh blade, bending the image so you see about 30° farther into the larynx. The image is right-side up. Knowing the exact location of the larynx helps aim the endotracheal tube (Fig 12-6). The prism will fog if not warmed beforehand — easily done by immersion in hot water or storage in your pocket.

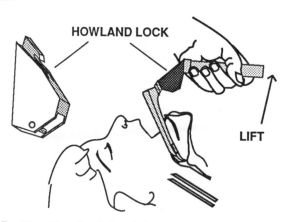

Fig. 12-5. The Howland Lock increases the angulation of the blade and improves mechanical advantage.

Flexible Fiberoptic Bronchoscopes

Many anesthesia services and intensive care units use fiberoptic bronchoscopes regularly for difficult intubations. Bronchoscopy is harder than direct laryngoscopy because bronchoscopes have several controls for manipulating the angle of the tip; because the narrow angle of view makes interpretation of the image more difficult; and because they are awkward to hold while maneuvering the tube.These instruments often cost in excess of $500 and are easily damaged if you ignore certain precautions.

The device consists of a long cable containing bundles of thread-like glass fibers connected to a pistol grip handle holding the control knobs. The handle attaches to a portable light source by another long cable (Fig. 12-7). Light travels down the glass bundles with minimal loss in brightness because of the internal reflection within the glass threads. The image returns along the same route.

Since the fiberoptic bundles are glass, *never* bend the cables or wrap them tightly around your hand. Holding the cable in a single *loose* coil avoids breakage. Don't pile equipment on top of the scope. Train anyone who has to clean the scope how to avoid breakage.

First, attach the light source. Look through the viewfinder and focus the lens by aiming the tip at some printed text. Note the distance of the object from the tip of the cable when the image focuses. Hold the lens cable straight and gently turn the control knob. Memorize which way the cable curves when you turn the knob (Fig. 12-8).

The unprepared lens will fog. Warm it to body temperature by immersing the tip in warm water. Apply an antifogging solution. A dab of mineral oil or antifogging soap works well. Use hibiclens if antifog-

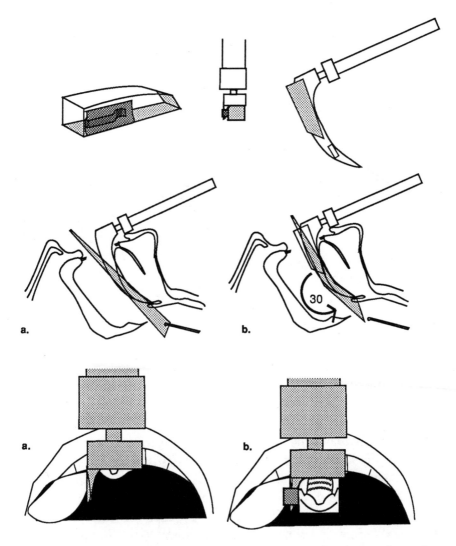

Fig. 12-6. The Huffman Prism brings an anterior larynx into view.

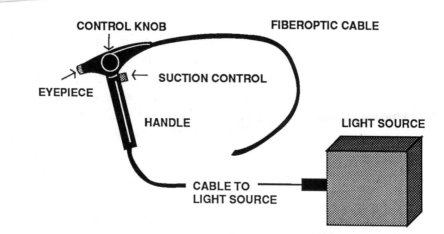

Fig. 12-7. The fiberoptic bronchoscope.

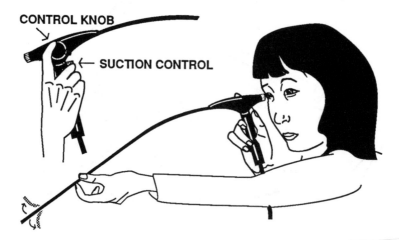

Fig. 12-8. Practice with the controls *before* inserting the bronchoscope.

ging soap is not available. Dry the lens tip carefully to avoid scratching it.

Choose the largest tube you can as this eases cable insertion and avoids damage. Too small a tube may wrinkle the cable's plastic covering. On the other hand, a pediatric cable may not be stiff enough to guide a large tube. An adult scope will fit any tube 6.5 mm (26 Fr.) or larger. A pediatric scope will fit inside a 4.5 mm (20 Fr.) or larger tube. Lubricate the cable with K-Y jelly or lidocaine ointment by spreading lubricant with a gauze pad from a point 2.5 cm (1inch) from the tip back toward the handle. Lubricant on the lens will blur the image.

Fiberoptic bronchoscopy allows intubation of both conscious and unconscious patients. Awake intubation lets patients breathe and protect their own airway.

Use a nasal vasocontrictor with nasal intubations to reduce the risk of nose bleeds (see Chapter 9). Give your patients atropine or Robinul to dry their oral secretions. Both treatments take several minutes to work so give the medication ahead of time — if possible. Suction the airway frequently during the intubation. Instrumentation of the oropharynx, sedation, and local anesthesia of the airway predispose to aspiration — *even though your patient is awake.*

I usually stand at the head of the bed to intubate with the fiber–optic bronchoscope (Fig. 12-9a). This is easier for me because I find it easier to visualize the anatomical relations in the standard intubating position. You can also stand at the patient's side facing the head (Fig. 12-9b). When standing to the side, reverse your directions for controlling the tip. From the side, aiming toward the patient's left means turning the cable tip to *your* right. Aiming anteriorly means turning the tip down instead of up. A short intubator may prefer to stand on a stool. Hold the cable in the left hand and the pistol grip in the right, using either your right thumb or index finger to turn the control knob. Keep the cable fairly straight. Dimming the room lights slightly may improve your image — if lower lighting doesn't compromise patient safety.

For oral intubation, insert the scope into the endotracheal tube and slide the tube toward the handle. This gets it out of your way. Put the cable into the patient's mouth. Have the patient stick his or her tongue out or have your assistant gently pull the patient's tongue forward. Advance the cable while looking into the eyepiece. Identify structures as you see them (Fig. 12-10). Flex the tip anteriorly to see the larynx. Make certain the tip isn't in the tube when you flex it or the threads may break. If necessary, to improve the aim rotate the distal end of the endotracheal tube. Pass the lens through the vocal cords when you see them. However, return the tip to neutral position before you advance it down the trachea. The image blurs during the passage through the vocal cords. A clear image of the tracheal rings appears on the other side and you'll see the carina if you advance far enough.

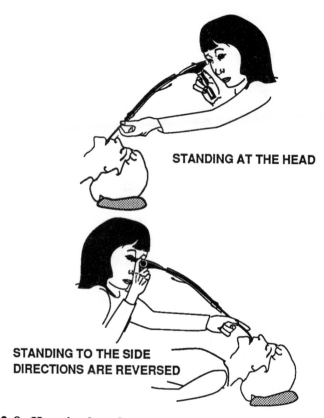

STANDING AT THE HEAD

STANDING TO THE SIDE
DIRECTIONS ARE REVERSED

Fig. 12-9. Keep back and arm straight for bronchoscopy positioning.

Hold the instrument steady and slide the tube down the cable using it as a guide. If the tube won't pass, rotate it gently to allow the tip to slide off the anterior commissure. Remove the cable, attach your 15 mm adapter and oxygen source, and ventilate. Check breath sounds.

Oral intubating airways help placement by guiding the tip of your cable in the general direction of the larynx. They also keep the patient from biting your expensive instrument or fingers. Anything leading to the base of the tongue guides you to the larynx; for example, a MacIntosh blade held by your assistant. Simply follow the curve with the tip of the cable.

With dimmed room lights, you'll actually see the light shining through the neck as the tip nears the larynx. As the cable enters the trachea the light moves down toward the chest and disappears. Failure

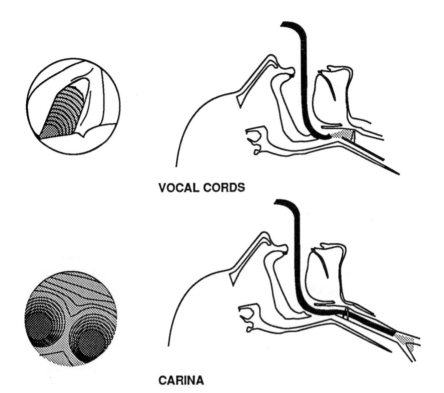

VOCAL CORDS

CARINA

Fig. 12-10. Viewing the larynx and trachea with a the fiberoptic bronchoscope.

to see the light as the cable advances may mean esophageal placement.

Inability to identify landmarks may mean the scope lies in the esophagus. Pull the cable back until recognizable landmarks appear. You'll see a grey tunnel with the lens inside the tube.

For fiberoptic nasal intubation place the endotracheal tube into the posterior pharynx before inserting the bronchoscope cable. The tube is more flexible this way and turns the corner more easily. Advance the tube until it just enters the posterior pharynx, then stop. Placing the endotracheal tube opening near the larynx often positions the tip of the bronchoscope below it. You may not recognize landmarks. When you do, the extreme angle that the scope must turn to reach the larynx may prevent entry through the vocal cords. Passage through the nose sometimes bends the endotracheal tube and may prevent insertion of the cable. Good lubrication and slight reposition-ing of the tube often cure this problem.

Rarely, the fiberoptic will pass through the Murphy Eye in the posterior pharynx and prevent intubation. Check for this if your fiber-optic is clearly in the trachea and you can't insert the tube.

Always use gentle technique. It's often better to start with the fiberoptic bronchoscope whenever you think you might eventually need to use it. Multiple prior attempts at blind intubation may bloody the airway and make identification of structures difficult.

You can ventilate with a nasal airway plus endotracheal tube adapter (Fig.12-11). An assistant ventilates while sealing the mouth and nares around the instrument. This technique can be used on apneic patients and also to maintain deep anesthesia during intubation under general anesthesia. Always have someone verify ventilation by listen-ing to breath sounds. Don't rely on chest movement alone. After intu-bation, suction the endotracheal tube to remove secretions or blood.

Use of the fiberoptic bronchoscope requires practice and emer-gencies are a poor time to learn the skill. Practice intubating the man-nikin with the fiberoptic if you have one. Anesthesia and surgical personnel can use it during routine intubation of patients with normal airways scheduled for elective surgery.

Retrograde Wires

A wire or catheter — passed through the cricothyroid membrane and advanced up into the oropharynx— can act as a guide for the endotra-cheal tube. You may perform the procedure with the patient awake or asleep. Only use this method if you can ventilate the patient during the intubation, because it takes several minutes to perform. When you can't ventilate, an emergency cricothyroidotomy or tracheostomy makes more sense. Contraindications include coagulation abnor-malities, extensive subglottic tumor growth, inability to identify the cricoid membrane due to tumor, skin infiltration, or scar tissue.

Identify the cricothyroid membrane and clean the skin with anti-septic. If time and patient condition permit use transtracheal lidocaine (see Chapter 13) after a skin wheal of lidocaine with epinephrine to

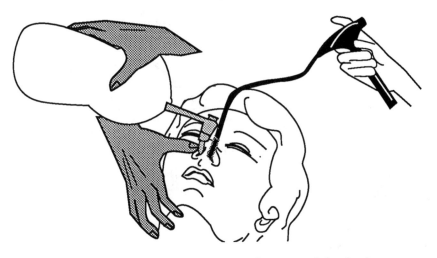

Fig. 12-11. Ventilation with a nasal airway and Ambu bag .

reduce skin bleeding. The guide catheter must be long enough to pass up the trachea, out the oropharynx, and then through the entire length of an endotracheal tube. A 0.035 cm ga. 145 cm vascular guide wire works well when passed through an 18-14g IV catheter. Other choices include a self-contained long-line CVP kit, or an epidural needle and catheter. Any wire should have a soft, flexible tip if possible.

Attach your IV cather or needle to a syringe and aim the bevel toward the patient's head. Aspirate air as you enter the trachea through the cricothyroid membrane and then hold the needle firmly. Detach the syringe and thread the wire through the IV catheter (Fig. 12-12). The wire will usually pass out the mouth or nose although it can go down to the carina or coil in the posterior pharynx. Use Magill forceps to pull the wire when you see it. Have an assistant firmly hold the end of the wire. Be gentle to avoid trauma or pneumothorax.

For oral intubations, pass the wire through the Murphy eye from *outside* in. Push it up the tube until it exits at the top. Hold the wire tense. Slide your endotracheal tube down the wire. The tip should enter the larynx and stop when the Murphy eye is level with the catheter's entrance hole and the tip is about 2 cm below the vocal cords. Hold the tube securely, pull the wire out of the tube from below, and advance the tube down the trachea. Check proper placement.

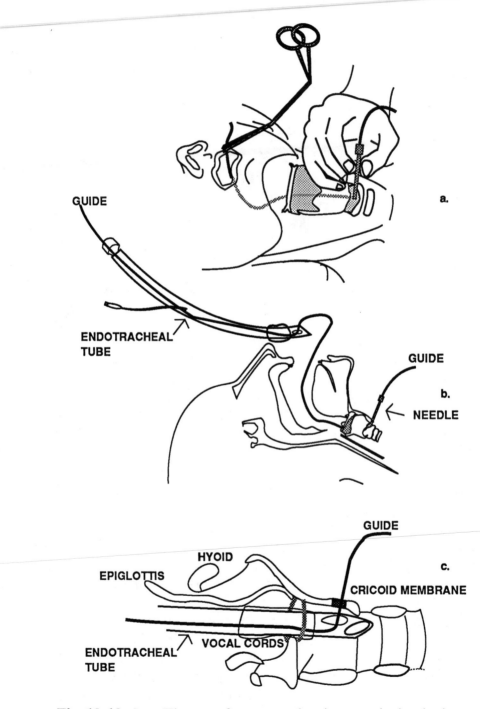

GUIDE

ENDOTRACHEAL
TUBE

a.

GUIDE

b.

NEEDLE

GUIDE

HYOID

EPIGLOTTIS

c.

CRICOID MEMBRANE

VOCAL CORDS

ENDOTRACHEAL
TUBE

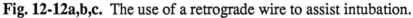

Fig. 12-12a,b,c. The use of a retrograde wire to assist intubation.

Sometimes the guidewire will pass out the nose on its own. If it doesn't — and you desire a nasal intubation — pull the guidewire through the mouth as described. Pass a cut NG tube or large bore suction catheter through the nose into the posterior pharynx and out the mouth. Pass the wire up through it and out the nose. Insert the guide catheter into the lumen of the endotracheal tube and advance the tube into the trachea. In this situation, the tip of the endotracheal tube will lie level with the catheter's entrance hole, about 1 cm below the cords. Hold the tube securely, withdraw the wire, and advance the tube. Again, check proper placement.

You can make the guidewire stiffer by threading it through an endotracheal tube exchanger or Eschman stylet preloaded with an endotracheal tube.

Combining Anterograde Fiberoptic Bronchoscopy With a Retrograde Wire

You can take advantage of both techniques to make intubation easier and faster. First, place a 0.035 cm ga. 145 cm diameter retrograde wire through the cricothyroid membrane and advance it into the oropharynx as described above. Insert your fiberoptic inside your endotracheal tube, then thread the guidewire into the fiberoptic's suction channel until the wire exits the channel near the eyepiece. Pull the guidewire rigid as you advance the fiberoptic/tube combination into the trachea. Remove the wire from below and insert the fiberoptic deeper into the trachea. Pass your endotracheal tube over the fiberoptic, then verify placement by listening to breath sounds.

Rigid Bronchoscopy

Intubation with a rigid bronchoscope sometimes works when all else fails. Improper use can cause severe trauma, so I don't recommend them for individuals not specifically trained in their use.

Surgical Cricothyroidotomy

Chapter 10 describes needle cricothyroidotomy as a quick way to give oxygen to the patient with airway obstruction. Surgical cricothyroidotomy is more hazardous. Consult an experienced surgeon to perform or to assist you with this procedure unless a delay will jeopardize patient survival.

Find the cricoid membrane and prep the skin. Use local anesthesia if you have time. Pull the skin tight and make a shallow incision over the cricoid membrane. Dissect bluntly and rapidly down to the membrane (Fig. 12-13a). Take care to avoid the large superficial veins and the thyroid gland. Cricothyroidotomy is fairly bloodless if you don't damage these vessels.

Make a stab wound about 1-1.5 cm long in the cricoid membrane with a number 11 blade. Twist the blade to allow ventilation (Fig. 12-13b).

Pull the cricoid ring upward with a tracheal hook or a clamp. This opens the trachea and allows insertion of a tracheostomy or endotracheal tube (Fig. 12-13c). If the incision is too small, use curved scissors or a tracheal dilator to *bluntly* spread the opening. Check breath sounds immediately to make sure your tube lies in the trachea and not the subcutaneous tissue.

Potential complications from this emergency procedure include injury to the larynx, hemorrhage into the trachea, aspiration, pneumothorax, esophageal damage, and subcutaneous or mediastinal emphysema. *Death* from asphyxia — from failure or from improper placement of the tube — can also occur. Use surgical cricothyroidotomy with great care.

Due to the greater complexity of the surgery and the increased risk of complications tracheostomy is beyond the scope of this book.

Further Reading

Guggenberger H, Lenz G: Training in Retrograde Intubation. Correspondence. *Anes* 1988; 69:292.

Lechman M, Donahoo J, MacVaugh H: Endotracheal Intubation Using Percutaneous Retrodrade Guidewire Insertion Follwed by Anterograde Fiberoptic Bronchoscopy. *Crit. Care. Med.* 1986; 14: 589-560

Patil V, Stehling L, Zauder H :*Fiberoptic Endoscopy in Anesthesia.* Chicago-London. Year Book Medical Publishers.

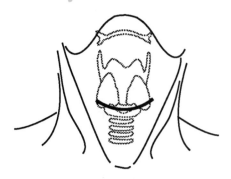

a. **MAKE TRANSVERSE INCISION THROUGH SKIN. DISSECT RAPIDLY DOWN TO CRICOID MEMBRANE.**

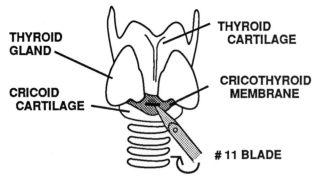

b. **MAKE STAB WOUND IN CRICOID MEMBRANE WITH #11 BLADE. TWIST BLADE TO ALLOW VENTILATION.**

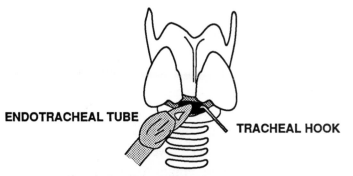

c. **PULL CRICOID RING FORWARD WITH HOOK OR CLAMP. INSERT ENDOTRACHEAL TUBE.**

Fig. 12-13a.b.c. Surgical cricothyroidotomy.

13

Awake Intubation
Increasing Comfort

G ood sedation reduces anxiety, speeds intubation, and often induces amnesia for a potentially unpleasant procedure. Local anesthesia also increases the comfort and ease of intubation. However, their use carries some risk.

Risks of Using Sedation

Under-sedation — Possible direct consequences include: poor cooperation raising the risk of trauma and aspiration; difficulty performing the intubation; hypertension and tachycardia; psychological trauma to the intubator; a poor evaluation of the medical care delivered.

Over-sedation — Over-sedation, however, can be more dangerous than under-sedation. Potential complications include: uncontrolled general anesthesia; hypoventilation (hypercarbia, hypoxia, apnea, cardiac arrest); decreased protective airway reflexes: aspiration; disorientation: poor cooperation.

Describing the intubation in *understandable* language reduces the need for sedation or anesthesia. Reassurance during intubation further reduces fear. "Hand holding" often works better than valium.

Learning to sedate properly takes practice. Always start with small doses and determine their effect before giving more. Table 13-1 lists common drugs and typical starting doses. Avoid the tendency to sedate heavily to make yourself feel more comfortable. As you gain skill you can often, *but not always*, predict the effect in advance.

We use two basic types of sedatives: hypnotics and analgesics. Hypnotics, such as valium, midazolam, or droperidol cause sleep and decrease anxiety. They often produce amnesia. Narcotics such as morphine, fentanyl, and demerol give analgesia, although they also add sedation. To treat anxiety, use a hypnotic. To treat pain, use a narcotic.

Factors Influencing Drug Effect

Drug potency, dosage, route, and speed of administration— Giving larger doses or more potent drugs will increase sedation. Giving the medication very slowly reduces this effect. As a rule, intravenous drugs sedate more than intramuscular drugs, because levels in the brain rise more rapidly.

Previous drug exposure — Patients who drink heavily or who use narcotics or tranquilizers regularly need more sedation.

Pre-existing sedation— An already sedated patient needs less drug to lose consciousness. This is true even if he doesn't appear sleepy at the time. Potential causes for pre-existing sedation include:

- other drugs
- alcohol
- hypoxia
- hypoglycemia
- exhaustion
- hypothermia
- hyperthermia
- electrolyte or acid/base imbalances
- malnutrition
- shock
- hypercarbia

Age — Elderly patients and children need less drug for sedation.

Pre-existing disease — Renal or liver failure may alter metabolism or excretion of sedatives, increasing their effect.

Emotional state — Fear increases the tolerance for sedatives. Be careful, however. After the intubation the now calm patient may lose consciousness and become apneic. Sedatives also release inhibitions. A previously stoic patient may become uncooperative after a sedative.

Pain — Pain decreases the effectiveness of your sedatives. Once the discomfort is gone, the sedatives may suddenly take effect.

Diurnal rhythm — In my experience, it's easier to sedate patients at night than during the day. They often sleep longer once sedated.

Evaluating the Effect of Sedation

To judge the need for further sedation, evaluate the following.

Will the patient tolerate any sedation? Avoid sedation in shock, airway obstruction, or respiratory failure, unless it's absolutely necessary. These patients may become apneic, hypotensive, or obstruct their airways with small amounts of sedation.

Is this patient at risk for aspiration? Sedate lightly when there is risk of aspiration. Always have suction available and watch the patient.

Will sedation make the intubation safer? Patients with hypertension or angina need stress reduction. Struggling patients may injure themselves. Alert patients guard their airways more forcefully.

What is the emotional state of the patient? Calm, cooperative patients need little sedation. Fearful or belligerent patients may need a lot. Remember that hypoxia or hypotension cause restlessness and lack of cooperation. Rule these out before giving more sedation.

Is ventilation adequate? Check skin color, rate and depth of respirations, presence of breath sounds, and air exchange.

Careful medication and observation lets you use sedatives safely.

Local Anesthesia of the Oropharynx

Applying local anesthetics to the mucous membranes numbs them easily. However, such numbness is non-specific and hard to control.

Table 13-1. Suggested Adult Starting Doses for Intravenous Sedation

Drug	Intravenous Dosage	Advantages	Disadvantages/ Potential Side Effects
Valium (10mg/cc)	2.5-10 mg (0.035-0.15 mg/kg) give 1-2.5 mg increments	amnesia sedation minimal respiratory depression	thrombophlebitis long acting no analgesia no reversal
Midazolam (1,5mg/cc)	1-5 mg (0.01-0.07mg/kg) give 0.5-1 mg increments	amnesia short acting (1-2 hrs) no active metabolites minimal respiratory depression	no analgesia no reversal *6X stronger than valium*
Thiopental (25mg/cc)	25-75 mg (0.35-1 mg/kg) give 25-75 mg increments	amnesia very short acting (minutes) minimal respiratory depression *low dose*	antanalgesic hypotension disorientation no reversal myocardial depression
Morphine (10 mg/cc)	1-5 mg (0.01-0.07 mg/kg) give 1-2 mg increments	good analgesia some sedation reversed with narcan	respiratory depression nausea / vomiting
Fentanyl (50 µg/cc)	25-75 µg *(microgram)* (0.35- 1 µg/kg) give 25 µg increments	good analgesia reversed with narcan	minimal sedation respiratory depression
Demerol (50 mg/cc)	12.5-50 mg (0.2- .75 mg/kg) give 12.5 mg increments	good analgesia reversed with narcan	respiratory depression nausea / vomiting tachycardia dry mouth
Droperidol (2.5 mg/cc)	1.25-5mg (0.02- 0.07 mg/kg) give 1.25 mg increments	sedation antiemetic	dysphoria
Ketamine (10, 50, 100 mg/cc)	10-100 mg give 10 mg increments	dissociative anesthetic (0.15- 1.5 mg/kg) active airway reflexes	hallucinations amnesia bronchodilator increased secretions tachycardia / hypertension increased intracranial pressure

Injection of local anesthetics directly onto individual nerves anesthetizes quite specific areas of the pharynx and larynx. Such nerve blocks require knowledge of the anatomy and a recognition of the potential complications of each block. While I don't recommend them for the occasional intubator, they're valuable to the experienced intubator.

Internal Layngeal Nerve Block — The internal laryngeal nerve is a branch of the superior laryngeal nerve. It provides sensation over the laryngeal surface of the epiglottis, the larynx above the vocal cords, the vallecula, and the lower pharynx. It penetrates the thyro–hyoid membrane midway between the hyoid bone and the thyroid cartilage about 1 cm anterior to the superior thyroid cornu.

Pressing on the opposite side of the larynx makes the landmarks more obvious (Fig. 13-1). Clean the skin with antiseptic. Find the superior thryoid cornu on the block side. The carotid sheath lies beneath your finger and the internal laryngeal nerve lies in front of your fingertip. Insert a 25 or 26 g needle attached to a 3 cc syringe into the thyro–hyoid membrane. You will feel resistance when you enter the membrane at a depth of 1-2 cm. Inject 2 cc of 1-2% lidocaine at this point. If you can't feel the membrane, advance into the hypopharynx and aspirate air. Withdraw the needle slowly until you can no longer aspirate air. Your needle tip should now lie just inside the membrane. Aspirate before you inject to avoid intravascular injections.

A block here preserves motor control of the cricothyroid muscle.

To avoid injection, place small sponges or gauzes soaked in 2% lidocaine into the piriform fossae bilaterally for 3-5 minutes. *Don't forget to remove them.*

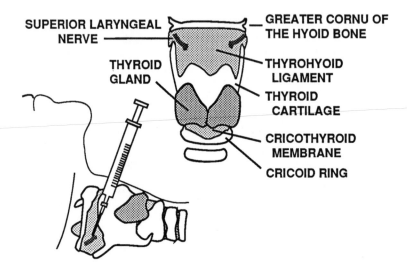

Fig. 13-1. Superior laryngeal nerve block.

Glossopharyngeal Nerve Block — The glossopharyngeal nerve gives sensation to the posterior third of the tongue, uvula, soft palate, and the rest of the pharynx. A glossopharyngeal block lets you insert an oral airway within about one minute without causing the patient to gag.

Although you can use a 22 g spinal needle to perform the block, a 23 g tonsillar needle makes the block easier and somewhat safer (Fig. 13-2). Depress the tongue with a tongue blade to stretch posterior tonsillar pillars. Insert the needle about 0.5 cm behind the midpoint of the posterior tonsillar pillar. Direct the tip laterally and posteriorly to a depth of 0.5-1cm. Aspirate carefully to avoid the carotid artery. A tonsillar needle has an angulated tip smaller than the rest of the needle to prevent deep insertion. Inject 3 cc 1% lidocaine bilaterally.

Combined internal laryngeal and glossopharyngeal blocks give excellent laryngeal anesthesia and depress the gag reflex. You may *cautiously* use them on patients with full stomachs because they preserve motor function. They preserve sensation below the vocal cords so any secretions or blood falling on or below the cords will still stimulate coughing.

Transtracheal Block — Transtracheal block provides anesthesia of the vocal cords, the subglottic larynx, and the trachea.

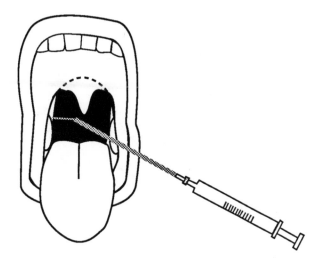

Fig. 13-2. Glossopharyngeal nerve block.

Insert a 23g needle attached to a 3 cc syringe through the cricoth-yroid membrane (Fig. 13-3) and aspirate air to check placement. Hold the needle firmly in your non-dominant hand and the syringe in your dominant hand. Inject 2 cc of 1-2% lidocaine rapidly and then quickly remove the needle. The patient will cough. Some operators use 25-26g needles. However, slower injection through the smaller needle means holding the needle firmly in place while the patient coughs.

A full stomach is a relative contraindication to transtracheal block. Maintain sensation below the vocal cords in this group if possible.

Acorn Nebulizers — Acorn nebulizers aerosolyze medications into the oropharynx and lungs, depositing a fine spray of droplets onto the mucous membranes and larger airways. We frequently use this device to treat bronchospasm. Aerosolyzing lidocaine will numb the entire oropharynx without injections.

Place 3-5 cc of 1-2% lidocaine into the nebulizer. Attach the nebulizer to your oxygen delivery system, such as a face mask. Wait until the liquid disappears, usually 15-20 minutes. By this time the pharynx, larynx, and trachea of the patient will be numb.

Complications of Local Anesthesia — Potential complications of injections include intravascular injection, bleeding into the airway,

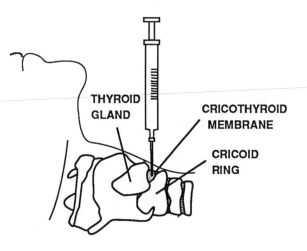

Fig. 13-3. Transtracheal nerve block.

hematoma, spread of tumor, and infection — although the risk of these is very low. Avoid airway blocks in patients with bleeding tendencies, infection, or tumor in the area of the injection.

Since oropharyngeal local anesthesia predisposes to aspiration guard against it. Always have suction available and use it frequently. Always suction the endotracheal tube after placement. *Never* leave the patient alone after numbing his airway, even if he seems awake and alert. Although aspiration can still occur despite all precautions, those precautions make it a very rare event.

Local anesthetic toxicity is a potentially serious problem. Calculate the cumulative total dose of local anesthetics *before* you use them. Don't give more than a total of 5 mg/kg of plain lidocaine or 7 mg/kg of lidocaine with epinephrine to your patient. Remember to add any local anesthetic needed elsewhere after the intubation.

Symptoms of local anesthetic toxicity are:

• sedation	• confusion	• tinnitus or
• metallic taste	• loss of	ringing in ears
• apnea	consciousness	• seizures
• arrythmias	• heart block	• cardiac arrest

Mucous membranes absorb medications rapidly. Don't let your patient swallow the local anesthetic. Instead, have him or her spit out the remaining liquid after holding the solutions in the mouth for several minutes.

If your patient shows signs of systemic toxicity then stop giving local, give oxygen, optimize airway and vital signs, and consider the use of valium to raise the local anesthetic seizure threshold.

Further Reading

Local Anesthesia

Barton S, Williams, D: Glossopharyngeal nerve block. *Arch. Otolaryng.* 1971; 93:186-188

Cooper M, Watson R: An improved regional anesthetic technique for peroral endoscopy. *Anes.* 1973;43:372-374

Gaskill JR, Gillies DR: Local anesthesia for peroral endoscopy. *Arch. Otolaryng.* 1966; 84:654-657

Index

About the Author

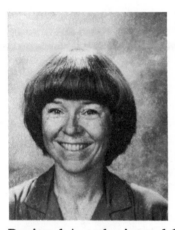

Dr. Christine E.Whitten is currently the Assistant Chief of Anesthesia at Kaiser Permanente Hospital in San Diego, California. She received her medical degree from Johns Hopkins Medical School in 1979. After her anesthesiology residency at the U.S. Naval Hospital in Portsmouth, Virginia, she completed fellowships in regional anesthesia and intensive care. Following training, she was on the teaching staff, Director of Regional Anesthesia, and Co-director of the Pain Clinic at the U.S. Naval Hospital in San Diego from 1983-1988. She became Board Certified in 1984.

Dr. Whitten is a co-author of "Anesthesia for the Developing Countries of the World" in *A Different Kind of Diplomacy: A Source Book for International Volunteers,* Plastic Surgery Research Foundation, San Diego, California, 1987. She is also the author of "Third World Medicine Is an Excellent Model for Operational Medicine," *Military Medicine,* (Nov. 1988), a series of 11 articles in *Emergency Medicine*, and instructor in a series of teaching videotapes on anesthesia techniques.

Dr. Whitten is an active volunteer for the international plastic surgery teams Operation Smile, Norfolk, Virginia and COAD International, San Diego, California. Both groups provide free surgery to children of less-developed countries. Besides participating in the surgical teams, she has also instructed anesthesia providers during these trips to Mexico, Vietnam, Honduras, the Philippines, Colombia, and Kenya.